HAVE FUN GETTING FIT

HAVE FUN GETTING FIT

Simple Ways to Rejuvenate Your Mind and Body

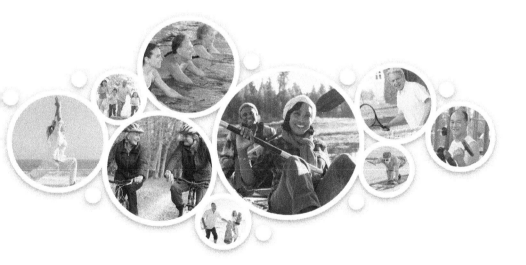

SHARKIE ZARTMAN

Dedicated to my husband, Pat, who has somehow managed to put up with me for forty-one years, which takes a lot of endurance! He is my best friend, soul mate, lover, and the strongest man I know, mentally, physically, and spiritually.

Contents

Acknowledgments

First, I want to give appreciation to the thousands of students and athletes I've taught and coached over the years, especially my new yoga students at the Anderson Senior Center in Redondo Beach, California. It's been such a pleasure and also a privilege to spend such quality time with incredible people who exemplify how important it is to share our talents and passions, enjoy life, and take good care of our bodies and health.

I've also been fortunate in having received a great deal of help in the development of this book from several people. My deepest gratitude to Martha Bullen, whose publishing expertise and knowledge have been guiding forces in this project. She is the main reason why I stayed on task. I am also grateful for Damian Fulton, who created the fun cartoons, Madalyn Stone for her excellent editing, and Jerry Dorris for the innovative cover design and interior layout. Also a huge thanks to Bruno Perron from SGI (Still Got It) and Dr. Tom Storer for their honest feedback and suggestions after reviewing the manuscript, and to my models, all over 60 years young, for letting me take their pictures for the book. They were so fun!

And last but not least, special thanks to my incredible dad, Len Boehnert, who at 93 years of age makes me realize that age really is just a number. He is the healthiest, happiest man I know who never takes any day for granted. One of his favorite sayings is "Every day above the ground can be a great day. Don't waste it!"

INTRODUCTION

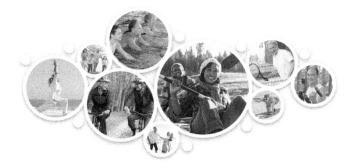

What if I told you there was a pill that helps people lose weight, increases muscle mass, elevates mood and energy, reduces stress, improves brain functioning, decreases the risk of most major chronic diseases, and also reverses the symptoms of aging—*plus* it has *no* side effects?

Would you take it?

Most of you would probably say: "Yes! Where can I get it, and how much does it cost?"

Well, I could make these pills easily. I would just get some vegetable capsules and fill them up with water.

However, the directions would say to take one pill fifteen minutes before exercising for at least thirty minutes every day. Take it once in the morning, and for faster results, once also in the afternoon.

Would it work?

For most people, if they followed this advice every day, they would assuredly see results.

However, it's not what's in the pill that is responsible for the results. It's the directions.

And the directions are to move your body every day.

When I give this example to the students in my health class at the college where I teach, they smile and shake their heads. Many of them don't exercise but do take a lot of pills. They just don't believe that exercise is really that important, although I am always on a mission to make them realize the value of having fitness in their lives.

For the students who do exercise, most of them are usually motivated by losing weight, getting muscle tone, playing their sport better, or looking hot in a bathing suit. Also, many of them exercise because it also helps manage their stressful lives.

However, as we mature, we aren't as interested in improving our sport or looking hot in a bathing suit anymore. Instead, we want to have mental clarity, be able to move our bodies without pain, and have enough energy to enjoy our lives to the fullest. We want to be able to play with our grandkids, travel, and make new connections. We also want to contribute to a greater cause and share our talents and experience with others. What we don't want is to end up feeble, be a burden on our families and society, or feel too old to do the things we want to do. Basically, we want to continue to have fun for the rest of our lives.

Well, I have good news for you! An active lifestyle might not guarantee these outcomes, but it certainly does give you the best opportunity to have the optimal life we all desire and deserve as the years go by. Obviously, people in the second half of life don't look exactly like they did in their twenties, but they still can do most of the activities they enjoy. It's like comparing a new car to a classic car; they both will get you where you want to go, but the classic car needs more care and might not get you there as quickly, but it will eventually arrive—with class!

Also, most active people fifty-plus feel between fifteen and twenty-five years younger than their unfit friends. Just take a look at the most vibrant, happy, fun people you know. Do they work out? Chances are the answer is *yes*! And even if they don't have structured workouts, they probably move a lot during the day.

As a professor of health and fitness at a community college for the last forty years, I have lectured, trained, and taught hundreds of fitness classes, thousands of students, and have experienced many trends over the years. I have also noticed that many of the students in my health classes really needed to so some physical activity, but when I asked them why they didn't exercise, many of them said that they didn't have the time, were too lazy, or it wasn't fun. Some even said that they didn't need it, which was not true after watching them try to fit into their desks.

Currently, I am also starting to notice a disturbing trend where many people use their age as an excuse not to do the things in life they desire and end up declining in health every year as a result. Trust me, I know firsthand that aging is definitely a challenge, but it is also an opportunity for us to finally follow our passion, and it is also a privilege. Just remember all the people you once knew who didn't make it this far.

I truly believe that as we get older, exercise is no longer optional if we really want to have a vibrant life all the way to the end. However, not only does exercise need to provide the results we desire, it must also be safe for our bodies, and for most people, has to be enjoyable. No one wants to exercise if it is viewed as punishment or something that has to be done—*or else*. I know I don't.

In this book, I hope to motivate you to find at least one or more fitness activities that you will enjoy and make a commitment to making them part of your lifestyle. Once you realize all the health benefits to be gained, why not give it a try? I am confident that the quality of your life can improve tremendously so you can enjoy your life to the fullest at any age. I am also on a mission to prove that the second half of life really can be the best half. Wouldn't that be cool?

In order to reach that goal, we need to respect and take care of our bodies and commit to being active each and every day. The rest of our lives are waiting for us. Let's *do* this!

CHAPTER 1

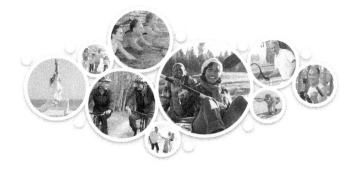

What Are the Benefits of Being Physically Active?

So why should you get active? What's in it for *you*?

First of all, your body is like an incredible machine that tunes itself up whenever you move. How much would you pay for a car that tuned itself up whenever you drove it? Our bodies were meant to move; however, many people spend too much time *idling*. In fact, we now have a name for that condition. It's called *Sitting Disease,* which is becoming more and more of a health concern because people are leading sedentary lives, especially from sitting at a desk working on their computers for long hours during the day.

In fact, some experts are saying that sitting too long, too often, is as dangerous to our health as smoking. My chiropractor also told me that he is treating many people with deformed spines and necks that have gotten that way from sitting all day and leaning forward at their desks and looking down at their computers. And these people are usually in their thirties!

The benefits of a fit lifestyle are numerous and available to anyone who is physically capable of moving. Alternatively, the costs of a sedentary life can strip away our quality of life and affect us both mentally and physically. So, if you want to live a dynamic life and get the best out of each and every day—*fitness is your best friend.* The choice is really yours. Do you want to be fit and vibrant or unhealthy and miserable?

If you are still reading this book, I hope you chose fit and vibrant.☺

Psychological Benefits of Exercise

What I love about the psychological benefits of exercise is that they are almost immediate. Research has confirmed the following major changes in psychological and mental health as a response to working out consistently:

- Decreases anxiety and depression
- Increases confidence and self-esteem
- Increases mental outlook
- Increases energy levels
- Helps develop a sense of control
- Improves sleep
- Improves memory
- Increases the ability to learn and concentrate
- Enhances creativity
- Relieves stress

If you ask a person who exercises as part of his or her lifestyle, "Why do you do it?" the response will most likely be, "Because it makes me feel great!" The reason for this can actually be attributed to the release of *endorphins*, the feel-good chemicals in the brain that activate its pleasure center. And who doesn't want to feel great?

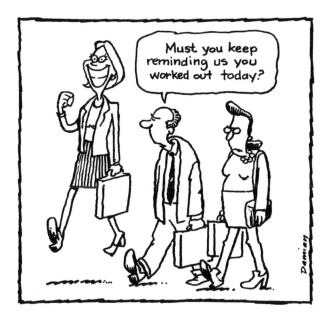

Weight Control and Metabolism Changes

Besides healthy eating, having a consistent exercise program is one of the best things you can do to control your weight and metabolism. It does take time to burn enough stored fat to make a change in body composition since there are 3,500 calories in one pound of fat. When you realize that an average workout only burns between 300 and 500 calories an hour, you can see why this is a long process.

Even though exercise burns very little fat during the exercise period, it has a tremendous effect on metabolism, or *basal metabolic rate*, which is how many calories you burn at rest. People who exercise as part of their lifestyle end up with more muscle mass, which needs more calories just to maintain. As a result, if you had two people sitting next to each other reading a book, one person could be burning almost twice as many calories as the other person if he or she had a high resting metabolism. Research[1] has also shown that caloric expenditure can remain elevated for up to seventy-two hours after exercising because of excess post exercise oxygen consumption. This is mostly true for resistance training and high intensity exercise.

Exercise also increases the fat-burning enzymes needed to break down stored fat into energy, which enhances fat burning even more.

Where does all this stored body fat come from? We can make body fat out of almost anything we eat. If we eat too many carbohydrates, proteins, or fat, our bodies will store the excess in the form of *adipose tissue*, which is actually stored fuel or energy.

Women store fat in certain places and men store it in others. The key to burning fat is getting the stored fat to move out of its storage site and go to the muscles where it will be burned for energy. Glucose is also used for energy and tends to be stored in the muscles and is burned first.

However, we want to burn the fat, don't we? Since fat is stored farther away from the muscles, it is a little harder to access when you start to exercise, but in a practical sense, it is inexhaustible. The key to burning fat is to exercise long enough to mobilize fat from its fat storage sites to be used for energy.

So how long does that take?

---

1   Borsheim, E. and Bahr, R. 2003. Effect of exercise intensity, duration and mode on post-exercise oxygen consumption. Sports Medicine, 33(14) 1037-1060.

For most people, at least twenty minutes of nonstop movement is required before the body *starts* to burn stored fat for fuel.

An exception is high intensity interval training (HIIT) in which the body switches between aerobic and anaerobic metabolisms or from high intensity bursts of exercise to low or moderate intensity. This is becoming a huge trend because it is challenging, fun, and doesn't take long to do. Also, there is an *afterburn* effect where the body burns calories after the exercise is over so you get even more fat burning for your time spent exercising. HIIT training obviously is intense, and you need to make sure you have healthy joints and also don't have any cardiovascular problems, such as high blood pressure, before you try this type of training.

Starting with slow, nonstop continuous training is safer for most people, but that doesn't mean that you can't add intervals on your own once your body gets accustomed to moving for at least twenty minutes.

After two or three months of steady exercise, the body starts to burn fat sooner in an exercise session, and this is especially true for women. The body is becoming *a fat-burning machine*. Also, as you progress and increase the intensity of your workout, you will increase your basal metabolic rate (BMR), mostly from increasing muscle mass, and burn more fat even at rest. Isn't that awesome?

So when it comes to losing fat with exercise, be patient. Losing fat is *not* hard. It just takes time.

Cardiovascular Benefits

In a study conducted in 2013 researchers found that higher levels of physical activity were associated with a 21 percent reduction in coronary heart disease for men and a 29 percent reduction of risk of coronary heart disease for women. The researchers concluded that higher fitness levels predict lower death rates and complications associated with cardiovascular disease. [2] This is *huge* when you take into consideration that heart attacks are the number one cause of death in the United States. When you take a look at all the cardiovascular changes that take place in the heart and blood vessels as a result of training, it is easy to see how these positive changes can prevent heart attacks.

The following changes occur in the cardiovascular system in response to a consistent exercise program where you move large muscle groups for at least thirty minutes a day:

1. The heart is able to pump a greater volume of blood with each contraction. This is called increasing the *stroke volume* of the heart.

2. As a result of the increased stroke volume, there is a reduction in the *resting heart rate*, meaning more rest for the heart between beats. This is energy saving for the heart. Consider the fact that an elephant can live one hundred years and has a resting heart rate of 25 beats per minute, whereas a mouse may live for only one year and has a resting heart rate of 600-700 beats per minute. The average human has a resting heart-beat somewhere in the 70s, but with endurance training, it could easily drop into the 50s and 60s.

3. Exercise enhances the development of collateral circulation providing an additional blood supply to the heart. This would provide alternative pathways should the coronary

2   Douglas Darden, Physical Activity and Exercise for Secondary Prevention, 2013

blood vessels supplying the heart become clogged. Also, existing arteries become larger and more elastic, enhancing blood transport.

4. Exercise also decreases the risk of plaque that contributes to *atherosclerosis* (narrowing of the arteries, which lead to heart disease) by clearing unhealthy cholesterol and triglycerides.

5. *High density lipoproteins* (HDL, the "good" cholesterol) increase with exercise. These particles may prevent the accumulation of plaque in the blood vessels, which is one of the main causes of most heart attacks.

6. A consistent exercise program may also prevent the rise in blood pressure that the average American experiences with increasing age. It can also decrease blood pressure in some people with chronic hypertension.

With all of these positive changes occurring as a result of exercise, it's easy to see how you could very well prevent a heart attack from ever happening or at least lessen its severity.

Muscle Benefits

Have you ever broken a leg or an arm and noticed how much smaller the limb was when the cast was removed? Disuse causes *muscle atrophy*, or shrinking muscle, and trust me, you don't want to lose muscle! Muscles need to be functional and strong in order for us to move.

Unfortunately, if you don't have an exercise program, your muscles will probably atrophy as you get older, and you will be less able to care for yourself physically later in life. Dick Van Dyke, the popular actor and dancer in the documentary, *If You're Not in the Obit, Eat Breakfast,* said that when he was in his 80s, he exercised to stay out of assisted living. Now he is in his 90s and can still dance and move with ease!

Also, remember that muscles move our body so we can get out and experience life! They are also where we burn fat for energy, so we want to keep them alive and healthy.

It is not necessary to become a body builder to keep your muscles functional, but adding some resistance training to your fitness program is vital as we age. Don't let those muscles atrophy!

Your Brain on Exercise

The most important parts of your body thrive on exercise. One of the most important organs is your brain. New studies suggest [3] that keeping physically active also keeps the brain active and might help prevent cognitive damage as we age. We now know that the brain actually makes new neurons and also new connections when stimulated by physical activity. Importantly, current research has shown that cognitive function and symptoms of dementia, even Alzheimer's disease, can be impacted with some types of exercise.[4]

So, if you are concerned about keeping mental clarity as you age, make sure you exercise every day to keep your brain cells healthy and nourished with oxygen and nutrients. We know that if we don't exercise, our muscles will atrophy or get smaller from a lack of activity; moreover, the same phenomenon happens to the brain.

---

3   Lytle, M.E. et al. (2004) Exercise level and cognitive decline: the 36 MoVIES project. Alzheimer Dis. Assoc. Disord. 18, 57–63

4   Larson, E.B. et al. (2006) Exercise is associated with reduced risk for incident dementia among persons 65 years of age or older. Ann. Intern.Med. 144, 73–81

The Benefits of a Adding Fitness to Your Lifestyle

Not enough to get you excited about working out yet? Well, here are eighteen other benefits of adding fitness to your lifestyle that are there for the taking. You might really like the last one.☺)

An active lifestyle:

1. Boosts the immune system, which helps protect against disease
2. Helps alleviate tension headaches
3. Improves heat tolerance
4. Increases the density of ligaments and tendons
5. Reduces the risk of adult onset diabetes
6. Along with diet, also helps to manage adult onset diabetes
7. May prevent osteoporosis
8. Improves balance, coordination, and may reduce the risk of falling
9. Protects against certain cancers, especially colon cancer
10. Slows the rate of joint degeneration
11. Helps to relieve constipation
12. Improves posture
13. Reduces work days missed due to illness
14. Improves the activities of daily living
15. Reduces health and medical care costs
16. Increases longevity
17. Improves athletic performance
18. Enhances sexual desire, performance, and satisfaction (Yes, seriously!)

◀◀ PEP TALK!

So, what's in it for you? In terms of overall well-being, developing an active lifestyle is the best thing you can do to feel great and have the quality of life you deserve regardless of age. Isn't that worth moving for at least thirty minutes a day? In a nutshell, a fit lifestyle will rejuvenate your mind and your body, give you more energy, and decrease the risk of chronic disease. Plus, you will be able to have more fun and hopefully never have to say, "I'm too old to do that."

CHAPTER 2

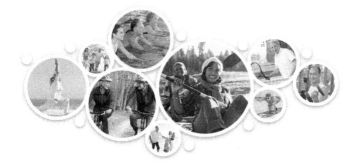

Understanding the Basics of Physical Fitness

I n a broad sense, *physical fitness* is usually defined as the ability to carry out daily tasks with vigor and alertness, without undue fatigue and with ample energy to enjoy leisure-time pursuits and to meet unforeseen emergencies. Basically, *physical fitness* is the body working at peak efficiency.

The exciting part about starting an exercise program is that you are never too old, too weak, or too out of condition to get benefits from exercise. Along with cutting your risks for diseases such as heart attacks, strokes, adult onset diabetes, certain types of cancer, and even dementia and premature death, an active lifestyle also increases the quality of everyday living. Simply stated, fit people have the capacity to enjoy life to the fullest. Isn't that enough of a reason to make it a priority?

Remember that you are never too old to do anything that you want to do. You might have a medical condition or injury, but for the most part, age should never be an excuse. I see many people in their eighties and nineties who are active and living life to the fullest. Plus, they are happy and fun to be around! For example, take Ida Keeling, who at one hundred years old, is the world record holder for the 60-yard dash. Her motto is: "I'm running from old age!"

In order to be physically fit, there are six necessary components. They are all important to understand and are also necessary ingredients to be at your physical best. They are: (1) cardiorespiratory endurance (sometimes called *aerobic fitness*), (2) muscle strength and power, (3) muscle endurance, (4) body composition (5) flexibility, and (6) balance. You can get most of these components in many activities, but you can also work on them separately. Once you understand the components and the principles behind them, you can plan your activities to get the most out of your workouts.

Component #1: Cardiorespiratory Endurance

Cardiorespiratory endurance is considered an important fitness component because it is *systemic*, which means it affects all body systems. It is defined as the ability of the heart, lungs, and blood vessels to deliver blood and oxygen to the working muscles and remove wastes during sustained activity.

The performance of moderately intense, sustained, large muscle group activities is the key to developing and maintaining an efficient cardiovascular system. Activities such as running, walking, swimming, skating, group exercise fitness classes, and dancing usually qualify as cardiovascular endurance exercises.

There is an ad on television about a medication with the message: "A body in motion stays in motion." I totally agree with that statement, but don't think that most of us need a pill to do that. And remember that there are a lot of activities that work the heart, so find the ones that you enjoy!

Component #2: Muscle Strength and Muscle Power and Component #3: Muscle Endurance

Muscular fitness includes muscle strength and muscle power as well as muscle endurance, and ideally, you should have all three.

Muscle strength is the maximal force a muscle or group of muscles can exert in a single contraction.

Muscle power is the ability to exert a maximal force in as short a time as possible, as in accelerating, jumping, and throwing objects.

Muscle endurance, on the other hand, is the capacity of a muscle or group of muscles to carry out repeated contractions without fatigue or hold a static position against gravity or resistance, for example, a forearm plank.

Exercises that focus on a particular muscle group, such as crunches for the abdominals or push-ups, and those that use resistance (such as weights, weighted balls, or tubes) qualify as muscle strength or muscle endurance activities.

When training for either muscle endurance or muscle strength, the difference involves resistance and *repetitions* (that is, how many times you lift the weights). For strength training, the resistance is usually high and the repetitions are low, whereas for endurance training, the resistance is usually low and the repetitions are high. For power training, the movements are performed quickly.

If you have good muscle fitness, you will have functional muscle mass that will make everyday activities much easier. Also, muscle is highly metabolic and burns a lot of calories, even at rest.

And remember that there are many ways to work with resistance, so don't do the same workout all the time. This not only stimulates the muscles to improve faster, but it also helps prevent plateaus and boredom.

Component #4: Body Composition

This component refers to the relevant amount of body fat as compared to lean body mass. *Lean body mass* consists of muscles, bones, nervous tissue, skin, blood, and organs, whereas *body fat* consists of adipose tissue, generally found below the skin (subcutaneous fat) and in the abdomen (visceral fat), which stores energy in the form of fat.

Your level of body fat can affect your risk of developing health-related problems. Too much body fat puts extra strain on your joints, impairs movement, and increases your risk of developing heart disease and certain types of cancer. Body fat, especially visceral fat, releases inflammatory agents that contribute to most chronic diseases. Too little body fat can also be a health risk and can interfere with the body's production of essential hormones such as estrogen.

Body weight alone is *not* a reliable indicator of body composition. A short, thin person could have a lot of body fat, and a tall, large person could have a large amount of muscle mass and very little fat. Therefore, we should be careful in interpreting metrics such as the *body mass index* (BMI) as an indicator of underweight, overweight, or obesity.

To determine body composition, there are three popular techniques including skin fold measurements, underwater weighing, and bioelectrical impedance. We'll talk more about these tests and how they are administered in chapter 9. For now, just know that the scale does not give any information on body composition. It only records total body weight, and from a health and performance standpoint, your body doesn't really care about how much you weigh. And remember that all activities burn calories, so when it comes to changing your body composition, find activities that you enjoy and be patient with weight loss.

Component #5: Flexibility

Flexible individuals can bend and twist with ease. *Flexibility* is defined as the ability to move joints freely through a full range of motion. Without routine stretching, muscles and tendons shorten and become tight as we get older. This shortening can impair our range of motion and make easy movements challenging and sometimes even painful.

The good news is that stretching is easy to do and will keep the joints mobile and prevent injury. Also, flexibility varies among the different joints in the body depending upon the structure and function of the joint. For example, the shoulder joint has a greater range of motion than the knee joint and can move in more directions.

Flexibility also varies in different people depending on their joint structure, age, fitness level, and gender. However, we still need to work on keeping our flexibility. If we don't, movement becomes restrictive, and our quality of life becomes impaired as a result.

Most people stretch before or after their activities, so usually it is easy to have flexibility as a part of your workouts. However, if you want to focus mostly on improving flexibility, there are several activities that will fit the bill, for example, yoga (see chapter 6).

Component #6: Balance

Some people consider this a secondary fitness component, but as we get older, balance becomes imperative for our functional health. Many people who have poor balance often end up falling and breaking their hips, which can obviously be a huge detriment to living fully.

Activities that include balance, such as yoga or tai chi or working with balance equipment such as stability balls, are fun and also challenging. Many people don't like to work on their balance because they are not good at it. But the good news is that they improve quickly, and that is always motivating.

General Fitness Principles

In order to see results from an exercise program, the activities should be consistent, progressive, and incorporate these general fitness principles: The FITT principle, overload, rate of progression, reversibility, and specificity. Trainers use these to make sure their clients get results, but once you understand them, you can use them on your own. The bottom line is that they work!

The FITT Principle

FITT is an acronym for:

    F = Frequency (how often)
    I = Intensity (how hard)
    T = Time (how long)
    T = Type of Exercise

By using the FITT principle, you can customize your workout to match your fitness level and goals.

Frequency. This refers to the number of times you participate in a physical activity per week. In order to maintain or improve cardiorespiratory endurance, authorities recommend ≥5 days per week of moderate intensity exercise or ≥3 days per week of vigorous intensity exercise or some combination of both ≥4 days/week. If you are trying to increase muscle strength or endurance, twice a week is enough to see results.

Intensity. *Intensity* is how hard you need to work in order to achieve a training effect or a positive physiological change as a result of exercise. Cardiovascular or aerobic training is usually performed at 60-90 percent of a person's maximum heart rate. A general estimate of your maximum heart rate is to subtract your age from 220. The resulting number is how much your heart can beat supposedly at full force.

For people who are in average to good physical condition, exercising at the 70-85 percent level will cause training effects to occur more quickly. However, exercising above the 85 percent range should only be done for short periods of time because high, extended intensity can cause soreness, fatigue, and also injury. However, short bursts followed by moderate activity appear to be safe for most individuals.

Time. This is also known as *duration,* and 30-60 minutes of continuous exercise is usually recommended for improvement in cardiovascular endurance. However, an accumulation of shorter exercise sessions can also cause significant benefits. Instead of working out for 30 minutes nonstop, some people show improvement from chunking up the time to three 10-minute sessions. This is desirable for people who don't have the time to fit in a full workout in one sitting. The emphasis is to try to get people as active as possible during the normal day.

Type. The types of activities that will improve cardiovascular endurance and burn fat are those that use continuous rhythmic activity of large muscle groups, such as running, cycling, skating, swimming, and various sports and high intensity interval training (HIIT). For muscle strength, power, and endurance, using resistance such as weights, tubes, machines, and even body weights are types of activities that will yield results. When it comes to choosing activities, go for the fun ones first! It makes working out a pleasure instead of a chore.

The following chart summarizes the FITT guidelines:

CV Endurance and Fat Burning for Body Composition	
Frequency:	3 times a week or more
Intensity:	60-90% of max heart rate
Time:	30-60 minutes ideally; 3 bouts of 10 minutes or more is also effective
Type:	Activities using large muscle groups that can be maintained continuously
Strength and Muscle Endurance (to get a combination of both in one workout)	
Frequency:	2 times a week
Intensity:	60-90% of one repetition max or a subjective rate of 5 on a 10-point scale of intensity
Time:	8-12 reps for most people, or for people over 65 years, 10-15reps
Type:	Resistance exercises that challenge the major muscle groups

Flexibility	
Frequency:	Minimum is four to five days a week
Intensity:	Stretch to a point of mild discomfort
Time:	10-30 seconds for each stretch
Type:	*Static stretching* (a held stretch) is the most popular and safest although *PNF* (involves both stretching and contracting a muscle group), *dynamic (slow controlled movement) and passive stretching* techniques (using an outside force to stretch, such as a partner or gravity) are also used. However, stay away from ballistic stretching (bouncing in and out of a stretch) because it might tear the muscle or the tendons.

These prescriptions can be modified according to a person's preference and current physical condition. They are just guidelines.

The Overload Principle

In order to continue to improve and maintain your training effects or results, once you have adapted to a workout level and it starts to feel easy, you must stimulate your body beyond its normal workload by either increasing the frequency, intensity duration, or by changing the mode of the activity. Too often, when adaptation occurs, people start to get discouraged because they are no longer seeing results. So make sure when your workout starts to feel easy that you change it up so you can continue to change and make progress which, in turn, will lead to more benefits.

Rate of Progression

So what's the time line as to when to expect results?

It really depends on the individual and the frequency, intensity, and duration of the activities, but generally speaking, there are three stages:

1. The first stage is the Initial Stage, which lasts about 4-6 weeks. During this time, you are adjusting to the physical demands of the activity. Starting slow and being consistent are keys to getting to the next step.

2. The second stage is the Improvement Stage, which lasts for 4-5 months. During this time, physical improvements become apparent; you are usually very motivated to continue.

3. The third stage is Maintenance, which usually begins after 6 months. At this point, the program should be evaluated to see if further improvements are necessary and if you need to change your routine.

Reversibility

You cannot store fitness. What a bummer! Just because you could run a mile in eight minutes a year ago doesn't mean that you can do it now. Detraining occurs in as little as two weeks following the cessation of exercise. This rate of decline depends on your level of fitness and the type of your activity. Remember this principle when you go on vacation. Make exercise a part of your life and an important part of your schedule. Hit-and-miss activity is not only ineffective, but it can be dangerous, especially if the intensity is too high.

Specificity

This principle is often ignored or misunderstood. However, it is one of the most important. Simply stated, *specificity* means that your workouts should match the physical demands of the desired result. For example, if you want to win a race, then you must increase the intensity of the workout, not the amount of time you exercise. Keep this in mind if you have specific goals. Design your workouts to help get the benefits that *you* desire!

PEP TALK!

You don't have to know these principles to get results. However, they are the nuts and bolts of understanding exercise physiology and fitness. Also, we are all different, and even if we did the same workout as someone else, we might not get the same results. We differ in many areas, including nutrition, age, gender, body types, muscle fibers, hormones, and our current state of fitness. We can all improve from exercise and get the perks, no matter what our fitness level or age might be, but they will not be uniform or equal in all people. And that is okay. So don't compare. Focus on what you are doing and stay active every day, and I promise the results will come!

You are really aiming to improve your quality of life by staying active and trying to have some fun while doing it. Your body is an incredible machine, and you only get one; it's not like a car that we can trade in for a newer version. But the great news is that the body regenerates itself with exercise, and you really can reverse the effects of aging with activity. Most of the problems and symptoms associated with aging are usually our bad habits catching up to us. So, how about practicing some new habits? Move every day and you will start to feel younger, more energetic, and happier. In case you're wondering, that's what's in it for *you*!

CHAPTER 3

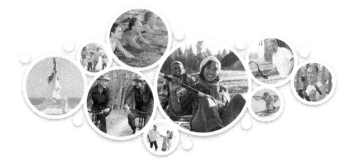

Getting Started

If you are just starting an exercise program or haven't exercised in a while and are ready to get active again, here are some suggestions to get your new fitness habit off to a great start!

The first thing you must do is GET YOUR MIND ON BOARD. As you probably already know, there is a huge mind-body connection. It's almost as if your body's cells are listening in on your thoughts. We need to make sure we have positive beliefs and attitudes before we get started.

Too often, people enter a fitness program with a fatalistic attitude. Messages such as, "I'm too old to do this" or "What's the use?" or "I tried exercising before and it didn't work" will sabotage even the best programs. Many of us have to clean out our heads and get into a positive mind-set. Here are some tips on how to do just that!

HOW TO DEVELOP A POSITIVE MINDSET

- Visualize your body the way you want to see it in the future and see yourself doing all the activities you want to enjoy.
- Experience the satisfaction and feelings of having a healthy, fit body.
- Start acting as if you have already reached your goal.
- Repeat positive affirmations each day, such as, "My body is healthy, strong, and relaxed."
- Seek out people who share your interests, support your goals, and are fun to be around.
- Keep your brain active by learning something new each and every day.
- Ask yourself, "What do I want to do with the rest of my life?" Let the answer be your motivation to stay active and fit enough so you can reach your goals.
- Don't focus on what you can't do; instead, focus on what you CAN do.
- Live your life and forget your age.
- Commit to being so busy loving life that you never realize you are getting older.
- Make your gift of time YOUR TIME to shine!
- Change your disempowering beliefs. For example, instead of viewing aging as an inevitable period of decline, view it as a challenge, an opportunity, and a privilege.
- Remember that a fit lifestyle is a journey, not a destination. Enjoy the ride!
- Focus on what you want instead of what you don't want. Positive expectancy is always a better way to move you

toward your goals. For example, instead of thinking, "I don't want to become frail and old," flip it instead to, "I want to remain vital and fit for the rest of my life."

Once you get your mind on board, the rest becomes easier. So check out what limiting beliefs might be holding you back from succeeding and change those beliefs!

There is an old Greek saying that fits in here: "Look for the good and you will find it. Look for the bad and you will find that, too." Remember that there is both good and bad in every person and every situation, and it's your choice as to how you want to view each situation in life.

Make Sure You Start Out Slowly

For most people, a fitness program should not pose any risk or problems as long and you don't try to do too much too soon. I have seen many students get excited on the first day of an activity class and try to keep up with everyone else but are so sore the next day they can hardly move. So remember to start any fitness activity slowly. Give your body a chance to adapt before you add more intensity.

Seek Medical Clearance if Necessary

It's always recommended to touch base with your doctor before starting any new exercise routine after the age of forty, especially if you haven't been working out regularly. While getting medical clearance to exercise is not necessary in most cases, if you answer *yes* to any of the following questions, you definitely need to check with your doctor before you start any exercise program:[1]

---

1   https://www.nasm.org/docs/default-source/PDF/nasm_par-q-(pdf-21k).pdf

THE PAR-Q PHYSICAL ACTIVITY READINESS QUESTIONNAIRE FOR SAFE EXERCISE

- Has your doctor ever said that you have a heart condition and that you should only do physical activity recommended by a doctor?
- Do you feel pain in your chest when you do physical activity?
- In the past month, have you had chest pain when you were not doing physical activity?
- Do you lose your balance because of dizziness or do you ever lose consciousness?
- Do you have a bone or joint problem that could be made worse by a change in your physical activity?
- Is your doctor currently prescribing drugs (for example water pills) for your blood pressure or heart condition?
- Do you know of any other reason why you should not do physical activity?

Personal Assessments

Whenever you go on a journey, it's always important to know where you are starting from in order to reach your destination. It's the same with fitness. The following are easy assessments you can do on your own in order to keep track of your progress. Trainers, coaches, and teachers can also have you do similar assessments for their classes or programs.

Besides tracking success, assessments can also serve as a motivation to keep you moving forward. You can track these in a notebook or journal.

1. **Take your resting heart rate.** Take your pulse for a full one minute either on your carotid artery or radial artery. The

carotid pulse can be found down from the corner of one eye just under the jawbone. The *radial pulse* can be found on the inside of the wrist on the thumb side. Use your middle and index fingers to feel the pulse. Don't use your thumb because it also has a pulse. If you find it difficult to take it for one minute, you can take it for thirty seconds and multiply by two. A normal resting heart rate is usually somewhere in the 70s. If yours is in the 80s or higher, it may come down as a result of your exercise training, and that is good! Remember that the less your heart has to work at rest, the longer your heart will supposedly last.

2. **Record your weight.** I know. Everyone hates to do this, especially those of us who have been avoiding the scale for a long time. But just do it this one time, record it, and forget it. You shouldn't have to record it again unless you want to for three to four weeks. Some of my students like to record their weight once a week or every two weeks—do whatever works best for you. However, I never recommend weighing yourself every day unless you are a masochist because weight can fluctuate a lot from day to day.

3. **Take your body measurements.** Using a measuring tape, measure these body circumferences and record:

    • **Abdomen**: At the level of the umbilicus (belly button)
    • **Calf:** The maximum circumference between the knee and the ankle
    • **Hips:** The maximal circumference of the hips or buttocks, whichever is larger
    • **Arm:** The widest area between the shoulder and the elbow

- **Waist:** At the narrowest part of the torso, usually above the umbilicus and below the ribs
- **Thigh:** The maximal circumference of the thigh, usually right below the gluteal fold

Record the measurements and then forget them for the next three to four weeks. What is cool is that sometimes the measurements can change dramatically without a change in your body weight. I once had a student who did not lose a pound during the semester but lost over 16 inches in her measurements. Obviously, she improved tremendously in body composition even though these changes didn't show up on the scale.

4. **Choose one cardiovascular assessment.** The ones we do at the college where I teach are usually either a 12-minute run or a mile test. If you are near a school that has a 440 track, you can easily do either test on your own. If you don't have a track nearby, you can set your own distance and be consistent about timing your progress.

- **12-minute test:** You will need a stopwatch for this test. On a 440 track, run-walk or jog nonstop for a total of 12 minutes. Record how many laps you covered to the closest quarter (4 ¼ for example). People who have good cardiovascular conditioning can usually get around the track at least four times in 12 minutes. Don't be upset if you don't come close to four laps in 12 minutes. Remember, whatever you achieve is a starting point upon which to improve. You are not competing with anyone else, so once again, record it and forget it for a while.

- **Mile test**: You can either do this on a 440 track or at a distance you know is approximately a mile. If you are on a 440 track, one mile is four laps. Again, record your time. If you are running or walking a set distance, let's say, from pier to pier or around a block, record how long it takes you to get from point *A* to point *B*. This test can be done anywhere. I do mine at the beach.

5. **Choose at least two muscle fitness tests.** The assessments usually used in a fitness class for muscle endurance are a push-up test, curl-up test, held plank test, and a wall sit. For a weight-training class, it is common to use a 1 RM test or a 10 rep max test. The 1 RM test (Repetition Max) measures the maximum weight you can lift on one attempt.

   - **Push-up test:** This measures muscle endurance in the upper body. It can be done either with straight legs or modified with bent knees. Remember to keep your back straight at all times. Record the number of push-ups you can perform in one minute.

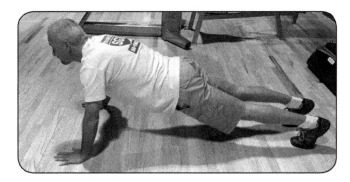

   - **Curl-up test:** Try to do as many curl-ups (crunches) as you can without stopping in one minute. Remember to keep your head in a neutral position and exhale on the way up. You can keep your hands on the floor or support your head with your fingertips as long as you don't pull at your head with your hands. Keep your knees bent. The action moves your rib cage toward your hips in a smooth, continuous action. If you prefer to do sit-ups instead, that is your option. However, most beginners can't do very many, so the curl-ups are a better option for many people.

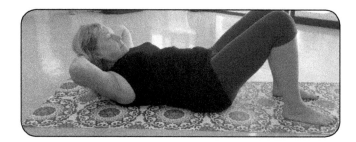

- **Forearm plank**: This one looks easy, but it's not. To get into position, start in the up position of a push-up, and then drop your forearms to the ground. Keep your hips level with your shoulders. Try to keep your body straight and hold the position for as long as you can.

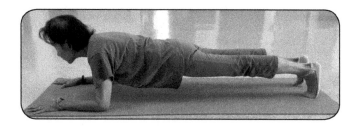

This assessment is great to measure core strength, which is much more than just the abdominals because it also challenges the back muscles.

- **Wall sit:** This test measures the strength and endurance of most of the muscles of the lower body. To do the assessment, lean back against a wall with your feet hip distance apart. Slide down to a sitting position as though you were sitting in a chair. Make sure your knees are right above your feet. Hold the position until you fail... usually when your legs start to shake. Trust me; it is harder than it looks!

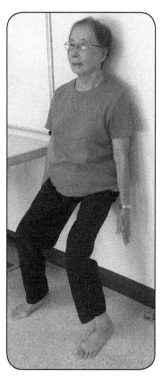

6. **Flexibility Test**

   - There are many flexibility tests, but the one I use most often in my classes is the Sit and Reach Test. It measures the flexibility of the hamstrings and lower back, two areas that are often very tight and can contribute to chronic low back pain.

   - To do the test, place a measuring tape between your legs while sitting on the floor with your legs straight at hip distance. The 0 mark is toward you and the 15-inch mark is at your heels. So when you stretch forward, if you can touch your toes, that would be measured as a 15. Anything less than 15 indicates less than average flexibility, and anything over 15 is better than average.

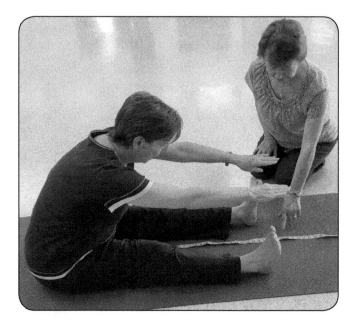

- I once had a student reach 28 inches. Obviously, she didn't need to improve anymore because her flexibility was almost superhuman. But most of my students either hit 15 or under, so they have a lot of room for improvement.

There you have it—six areas to assess before you start on your fitness journey. If you decide to do any of these assessments, I recommend that you retest every three or four weeks. Seeing results is fun and is also motivation to keep going!

You can also record your body mass index (BMI) and your blood pressure when you have your medical check-ups. They should be on your medical records, which are usually available online.

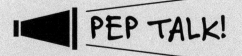

One of the most important things to consider before you go on your journey is where do you want to go? What are your goals? You know where you are now, so now is the time to ask, what do I want out of my fitness program? This is up to you and no one else. Your goals can be very general or specific. Write them down.

But remember, it takes time to see some of the changes you might be reaching for, especially losing weight, so be patient and enjoy the ride! However, most of the psychological perks are immediate, so let that be one of your goals—to feel good each and every day! That is achievable if you work out every day. Are you ready to get started? Let's go find some FUN activities!

CHAPTER 4

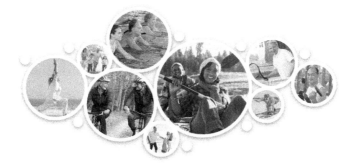

Finding the Right Workouts for You

This is where the fun begins! You get to explore fitness options, test out the ones you might want, and then work them into your schedule. It's like doing a taste testing before you order a meal.

If you like being around other people, take a look at group fitness classes. If you like to work one-on-one with an expert or in a small group, choose a personal trainer. You can also work out by yourself and use this time to just focus on what you want to do.

Group Fitness Classes

Group fitness classes usually have a lot of energy, and people support each other through the workouts. You can find them anywhere—at schools, clubs, YMCAs, and recreation centers. Some of the more popular classes are body conditioning, aerobic fitness, high intensity interval training (HIIT), boxing, cycling, boot camp, Zumba, body pump, sports conditioning, power core training, circuit training, and different types of yoga.

Most group fitness classes follow this progression: they start with a warm-up followed by the main event and then end with a cool-down. If time allows, there might be a period of specific muscle conditioning, and ending with a final stretch period. As you can see in this progression, most of the fitness components are included in the workout.

It's important to get to class before it starts so you don't miss the warm-up. Coming into a group fitness class late is not only rude, but it can also put you at risk for injury.

The intensity of the class can range from easy to extremely challenging. Make sure you find out as much about the class as you can before you sign up. Once there, *you* are usually in charge of your own intensity and can monitor it in three ways: heart rate monitoring, perceived exertion, and the talk test.

If you choose to **monitor** your **heart rate**, some of the classes will let you wear your own heart monitor. However, if they don't, or you don't have one and want to use this method to monitor your intensity, you can take your own heart rate by counting your pulse for 6 seconds, and then adding a zero (that is, multiplying by ten). If your heart rate is 11, then the exercise heart rate is 110. You don't ever want to get close to your maximum heart rate, which is 220 minus your age. That level would be very hard to sustain and could also cause injury. However, if it is a high intensity interval class, your heart rate can be high for very short periods of time.

Monitoring the intensity of your workout by **perceived exertion** is easier because it is subjective. You always know how you feel. It can be used independent of, or in combination with, your heart rate. *Perceived exertion* refers to the overall level of exertion experienced— the rate of breathing, muscle sensation, and the amount of effort.

When using the 20-point Rating of Perceived Exertion scale, you should exercise between an RPE of 12 and 16, or between light to hard. This usually relates to the theoretical heart range rate if you multiply the numbers by ten. If you want to check it out, take your pulse to see if your perceived exertion matches how hard your heart really is working. What's cool is that you will most likely find that your heart rate is roughly ten times the number you have chosen on the perceived exertion scale.

Rating of Perceived Exertion Scale

6	Nothing at all
7-8	Very, very light
9-10	Very light
11-12	Light
13	Moderate
14	Somewhat hard
15-16	Hard
17-18	Very hard
19-20	Very, very hard

If you chose 17 or very hard on the scale, your heart rate would be around 170.

The **talk test** is the easiest way to monitor the intensity of your workout. When you are exercising, you should be aware of your breathing and try to keep it rhythmic and comfortable. If you need to gasp for breath when talking between workouts, you need to slow down. Also, could you talk to someone else while you were working out? Or sing along with the music if one of your favorite songs were playing? These are other ways to pass the talk test.

There are several ways to slow down your workout intensity on your own should you need to do so. For example, if you are jogging, slow down to a march or a walk. If you are exercising with your arms raised above your head, drop them down below shoulder level or stop moving them and just move your legs. You can also shorten the range of motion and cut the movement in half. However, what you do NOT want to do is stop suddenly and sit down unless you feel dizzy or sick.

The instructor is usually directing the intensity at the mid-level of the class. If you need to turn down the intensity or turn it up, that's fine. Go at your own pace. But remember, this is supposed to be fun—not a grueling experience.

As far as choosing a class, go for the fun things first! Fitness has gotten so creative and instructors love to challenge their students and also mix things up to keep things interesting. So go into a class with an open mind and be ready for anything. Also, let your instructor know if you have any injuries or limitations.

Remember that there is no competition in a fitness class; people are not judging you, ever. However, there are some group exercise guidelines and tips that are important for you and the other participants to enjoy the class to the fullest extent.

DO:

- Make sure you bring a bottle of cool water and a towel.
- Get to class on time. Instructions are given at the start of

class. You don't want to be clueless as to what's going on because you were late.

- Begin slowly. Do not try to overdo. If you are late and miss the warm-up, do a warm-up on your own on the side or in the back of the class.
- Wear comfortable clothing that you can move in. In a fitness class, you do not dress to impress. Just wear functional workout clothes.
- Make sure you can pass the talk test during the main part of the workout. If you cannot talk or sing, slow down to a pace where you are able to.
- Make sure that if you have to leave class early, you cool down on your own in the back of the room.
- Make sure you have proper workout shoes. Many injuries can occur if you don't have proper footwear.
- Clear your mind of outside interference when you come to class. Be prepared to fully concentrate on the workout.
- Find a space in the room or on the field where you can hear the instructor.
- If you have any questions or concerns, ask the instructor. Remember, they are there for YOU!

DON'T:

1. Chew gum during the workout.
2. Participate in the class if you are sick or injured.
3. Ever push into the pain area. Pain is a sign that something is wrong.
4. Eat a heavy meal prior to class. Fruits, nuts, or juice are recommended snacks before class. Otherwise, allow yourself at least two hours to digest a normal meal before exercising.

5. Compare yourself to others. Remember, a group fitness class is NOT a competition.
6. Wear heavy perfume to class.

When working out with a group, this format brings a common sense of purpose, and most people enjoy working out with a group more than exercising by themselves. However, as a group exercise instructor for over forty years, I have seen many personality types in my classes. Some can present challenges, some are very positive, and others are just funny. All we ask as instructors is that you are considerate of others while participating in class.

Here are the ten most common personality types who participate in group fitness classes. Trust me, I have seen them all!

1. The **Gold Star Participants**: No, they are not the teacher's pets, but they are the students who keep us going. They are on time for class, listen to instructions, work at their own pace, are enthusiastic, smile, and will volunteer to either help the instructor or a fellow participant. These people are pleasant to be around, helpful, and instructors appreciate each and every one.

2. The **Exhibitionists**: These participants are overly concerned with how they look and how other people respond to them. They are usually stuck to the mirror or are positioned so that everyone in class can see their every move. These people are dying for attention. Just be nice and don't try to outdo them, or you will have a war on your hands.

3. The **Masochists**: These students work at 110 percent of their max. They must go higher, longer, and stronger than anyone else. You can always hear them moaning and

grunting. Too bad a fitness class is not a competitive event. They are risking their health to win a contest that exists only in their heads.

4. The **Effort Impaired**: These people are the exact opposite of the masochists. They don't' try at all. Getting these people to move any body part in any direction is difficult. They also are the ones who complain the most about not seeing any results. It is funny when an effort-impaired participant is working out next to a masochist.

5. The **Mighty Mouths**: These individuals move their jaws more than any other body part. At least you know that they can always pass the "talk test." They usually travel in packs and are most interested in gossiping than in any fitness-related activities.

6. The **Individualists**: These people feel they know everything about fitness and are not afraid to show it. They will sometimes do their own routines if they do not like what the instructor is doing, which is never appreciated. They will also gleefully point out when an instructor does more reps of an exercise on one side than on the other. We usually recommend that these people either get with the program, work out on their own, go to another class, or get instructor training so they can teach their own class.

7. The **Wrong Way Warriors**: Somehow, whenever the class moves in one direction, these people take off in another. They are not doing this on purpose like the individualists are, so instructors are more understanding. Usually, after an initial period of time, they get into the swing of things and are fine.

8. The **Clueless**: Nothing ever registers with these participants usually because they are not listening. For example, the instructor might have just given instructions on how to do an exercise, and the clueless will immediately ask how to do that very exercise.

9. The **Zombies**: These individuals never smile or react to anything the instructor says. The common expression on their face is a blank look. The instructor has to stifle a strong urge to take their pulse, just to make sure...

10. The **Escape Artists**: These people can't wait to leave the class, and as soon as the instructor turns his or her back, they are out the door. Sometimes they come back and sometimes they don't. We never know why they left (or even why they joined in the first place), so the whole thing usually remains a mystery.

Hire a Trainer

Not ready to work out with a group? If you are just starting a program and want to go at it alone, I would highly advise you to get a personal trainer to get you started on the right path. He or she will do assessments and design a program tailored to meet your needs and goals. Also, he or she will show you how to do the exercises correctly, which is very important, especially for resistance training. Finding the right trainer sometimes takes more than one try. You should want to go to your sessions and not dread them.

The trainer needs to be certified, and some of the best ones are found on NASM (The National Academy of Sports Medicine, www.nasm.org) and ACSM (The American Academy of Sports Medicine, www.acsm.org).

Make sure the trainer has experience working with people who are your age, have similar goals, or who have the same limitations, if you have any. Also, the trainer's personality is important. You don't want to pay for a babysitter who just counts your reps. The trainer should inspire you to stay on your program. Once you are on a path and know how to progress, you shouldn't need to keep the trainer. The trainer's job is it to train you to do your program on your own. It is NOT a long-term relationship.

On Your Own

There are a wide variety of workouts that you can do on your own. The choices are almost endless! However, there are a few things to keep in mind when you go at it on your own.

Walking

One of the best workouts that anyone can do, anywhere, is walking! And the best place to do it is outdoors! Most people don't consider walking to be exercise, but it is! Some of the benefits include:

- No new skills to master.
- It can be done anywhere.
- Requires no equipment other than shoes.
- Involves most of the body's large muscles.
- There is no injury risk.
- Enhances creativity and reduces stress.
- It can be done alone or with others.
- Burns between 300 and 400 calories per hour.
- Strengthens bones and may prevent osteoporosis.
- It is a great exercise for the overweight individual since it is easy to do and still burns calories.

Even though we all learned to walk at an early age, here are some tips that will keep you comfortable as you walk and also make it an effective workout.

1. Keep your posture tall! Do not bend forward.
2. Pull the shoulders back and keep them relaxed.
3. Pull the abdominal muscles in.
4. Keep your head and chin up and look straight ahead.
5. Relax your hands and swing your arms so that they brush past your body.
6. Keep your hips loose and relaxed.
7. You should land firmly, HEEL first. Roll from the heel to the ball of the foot and push off your toes and the ball of your foot.

One criticism people have when it comes to walking is that is can become boring. Here are some tips on how to keep a walking program fun and full of variety.

1. Walk in interesting places. A track, even though it is easy to estimate the distance, can get monotonous. Walk along the beach, in the parking lot around the school, or even in the mall. Start taking hikes through the mountains or hills and try new routes each time.
2. Walk with a partner or a group. Since you need to pass the talk test, this can be a great time to catch up on gossip, solve problems, or support each other.
3. For those who like solitude, think of your walk as a moving meditation. Move your awareness into the present moment and take in your surroundings with all the senses.

4. If you are walking in a safe environment or on a treadmill, try a headset or ear phones. You can listen to music or even learn a foreign language while you are walking. Time flies when you are listening to something interesting while you are working out.

5. Once you are comfortable with walking, experiment with intervals. For example, walk for eight to ten minutes, then jog for two to three minutes.

6. Sneak in walks whenever you can. Take a walk on your lunch break. Choose a parking place far away from the store instead of close to it. Take the stairs instead of the elevator or escalator. Find excuses to walk! Remember, you are an active person now.

7. For a challenge, walk hills.

8. Get a pedometer and have it count your steps. A standard guideline is to walk at least 10,000 steps a day. Most people only walk between 2,000 and 3,000.

Remember to progress slowly. Here is a walking program that will take you from a non-exerciser to an expert walker who can walk four miles in an hour. Do not go to the next level until you have adapted to the previous one. In other words, don't progress to the next step if the previous one was too hard for you. Wait until it is easy. You may start anywhere in the progression since the beginning levels are for very unconditioned exercisers. The times and distance are guidelines. They can be adjusted for individual needs.

Stage One: Getting Started

1. Walk briskly for 5 minutes. Rest or walk slowly for 3 minutes. Walk briskly again for 5 more minutes (total time: 10-13 minutes).

2. Walk briskly for 8 minutes. Rest or walk slowly for 3 minutes. Walk briskly again for 8 minutes (total time: 16-19 minutes).

3. Walk briskly for 10 minutes. Rest or walk slow for 3 minutes. Walk briskly again for 10 minutes (total time: 20-23 minutes).

Stage Two: Going the Distance (Use a 440 track if possible: 4 laps is one mile on the track.)

1. Walk 15-20 minutes nonstop. Distance covered: 1 Mile
2. Walk 20-25 minutes nonstop. Distance covered: 1 ¼ miles
3. Walk 25-30 minutes nonstop. Distance covered: 1 ½ miles
4. Walk 30-35 minutes nonstop. Distance covered: 1 ¾ miles
5. Walk 35-40 minutes nonstop. Distance covered: 2 miles
6. Walk 40-45 minutes nonstop. Distance covered: 2 ¼ miles
7. Walk 45-50 minutes nonstop. Distance covered: 2 ½ miles
8. Walk 50-55 minutes nonstop. Distance covered: 2 ¾ miles
9. Walk 55-60 minutes nonstop. Distance covered: 3 miles

Once you can walk three miles or more in an hour, you may want to consider integrating some short jogging bouts into your workout. If jogging is not for you, consider walking up and down hills, on soft sand, or even carrying hand weights to challenge yourself once you become an expert walker.

Most people do not automatically jump from being a walker to a jogger in one workout. However, the two exercise modes can be combined into a fun interval workout and also be progressed as a bridge from one mode to the other. Most jogging injuries come from doing too much too soon, which is the case with beginning exercisers who start jogging before their bodies are ready.

Here are two sample workouts that incorporate both walking and jogging into one workout. The first one is a slow progression, while the second one is a faster bridge. Your motivation and fitness levels determine which workout is the best for you. These are just examples. Modify and fine-tune them to fit your particular, individual needs.

The Beginning Bridge (walking-running intervals—2-3 times a week). All you need is a stop watch!

Segment	Time	Mode
1	22 min	jog 30 seconds, walk 5 minutes (4 times)
2	25 min	jog 60 seconds, walk 4 minutes (5 times)
3	27 min	jog 90 seconds, walk 3 minutes (6 times)
4	28 min	jog 2 minutes, walk 2 minutes (7 times)
5	27 min	jog 3 minutes, walk 90 seconds (6 times)
6	30 min	jog 4 minutes, walk 60 seconds (6 times)
7	33 min	jog 5 minutes, walk 30 seconds (5 times)

Gradually progress to continuous jogging.☺

The Intermediate Progression (continue mode for the assigned time)

Segment	Time	Mode
1	20 min	jog 10 steps, walk 10 steps
2	25 min	jog 20 steps, walk 10 steps
3	30 min	jog 30 steps, walk 10 steps
4	30 min	jog 1 minute, walk 10 steps
5	30 min	jog 2 minutes, walk 10 steps
6	30 min	jog 1 lap (1/4 mile) walk 10 steps
7	30 min	jog 2 laps with 10 steps in between
8	30 min	jog 1 mile (4 laps), rest with 10 steps, and repeat
9	30 min	jog 2 miles nonstop

You are NOW A JOGGER!

If you decide that you love jogging, make sure you have a good pair of running shoes. Since it is a high impact activity, however, jogging is not for everyone. A person who is carrying a lot of weight would be better off with a walking program or biking or swimming to prevent knee and hip problems because of the constant impact on the joints.

However, many people love jogging and the freedom it brings because it can be done almost anywhere. Also, there are many races that add extra motivation such as 5Ks, half marathons, and full marathons. I have seen some people who started a walking program, then advance to jogging, and are now racing in these events. These are some amazing transformations!

Sprinting

Doing wind sprints is one of the fastest ways to improve fitness and increase fat-burning enzymes. For overweight people, a sprint might just be a faster-than-normal walk that gets them out of breath. If an individual does this "sprint" two or three times during a 30-minute walk, the body responds by making more fat-burning enzymes. Also, there is an *afterburn* effect when the body burns more calories after the workout is done. You can throw in these wind sprints anytime during a walk or jog. They are fun and keep your workouts challenging. Think of them as *speed play*.

Interval Training

Athletes have used this type of training for many years, and it most recently has been added to group fitness classes as an alternative to a continuous intensity level. Interval Training is a fun and challenging group class that is becoming very popular. This is a great solution for people who complain that they do not have enough time to get in shape or for people who are frustrated from a lack of results. Most of these classes are identified as HIIT, although Cross Training classes also usually include intervals.

Interval training allows the body to adjust to more intense workloads by alternating them with lighter exercise bouts or rest periods.

This type of training is cool because you get results faster in less time. These workouts are usually shorter and work well into anyone's busy schedule. However, they are very intense and not recommended for people who have health issues.

Soft-Sand Training

I have to admit, this is my favorite, and I do it most mornings. We live close to the beach, and the soft sand is out there just calling my name. If you live close to the beach, why not give it a try? It is one of the toughest workouts you can do with the least amount of shock. Sand looks so harmless, and most of us view it as something we wipe off our bodies after we go to the beach. But if you are serious and ready for both a change in your workouts and also a challenge, give it a try. At first it will be hard, but you will eventually adapt and get tremendous benefits as a result. Walking, jogging, and interval programs can be done in the sand. Also, when you are done, you can just take a dip in the ocean!

Here are some guidelines on how to make sand work for you:

1. All sand is not alike. The sand closest to the water is the most hard packed, depending on the level of the tide. For beginners, start close to the water where the sand has some "give," but not enough to feel like quicksand. Make sure

the shore is even and not on a slant or your weight will be unbalanced. Check the tide charts in the paper to see when it is low tide. Anything under 0 is usually favorable to run close to the water.

2. Shoes are recommended, but many sand runners prefer to run barefoot. I know I do! Actually, the ankles and toes get stronger if you do not wear shoes, but then you have to watch out for glass, rocks, shells, and crabs.

3. When you are ready for the deep sand, move back from the shore and run or walk in the soft stuff. At first it might feel like you are moving in place since you will sink with every step. A nice alternative and bridge between the hard-packed sand close to the water and the soft sand is to find a tire track which still absorbs shock but is easier to run in because you don't sink as deeply into the sand. The next time you are at the beach, you might notice how many people are running or jogging in the tire tracks. It's great to get on one before anyone else!

4. Get some variety. You can run on hard-packed sand and then either do intervals or challenge yourself in the soft sand. Also, if you can find a sand hill, you are in for a real treat, because that is one of the most challenging workouts you can try.

5. At the end of your workout, sit down by the water, stretch, and look at the ocean. Then close your eyes and enjoy your surroundings. If it is a warm day, finish off your workout by taking a dip in the ocean! I always wear my bathing suit under my clothes and have a towel on the beach.

Don't live by the beach? There is a tremendous new training device called the Sand Dune Stepper (www.sanddunestepper.com) that mimics the action of soft sand. It is a soft platform that is used to improve motor skills; core, balance, and cardiovascular endurance; and weight control. It is also great for rehab and working the internal muscles of the foot. Plus, it is shock absorbent so it is safe for the joints. Several hospitals on the West Coast are now using the device for their patients. Therefore, if you want to simulate soft-sand training, this could be a great training device to have in your home.

Biking

Bicycling is an excellent aerobic activity for all ages and especially good for overweight and unfit people or those who might have leg or foot problems caused by impact activities. The only problem is finding a safe area to bicycle. You must also maintain your bike and in most places wear a helmet.

Also, be aware that the traffic stop signs and red lights also apply to bicyclists. I see many bikers go through these signs like they are exempt, and that's when accidents occur. For those who don't want to hassle these inconveniences, stationary biking is a great option. You can do this yourself at home or at the gym.

Also, if you haven't tried a spinning class, these are fun, challenging workouts although make sure you don't work out too hard and end up in the emergency room.[1] This can be a real concern especially for first timers who want to keep up with the class.

There are now also some places where the bikes are under water

---

1   Young, I. and Thomson, K. **Spinning-induced rhabdomyolysis: a case report.** *Eur J Emerg Med.* 2004; 11: 358–359

so the workout is even more challenging because you have to move your legs through the water. If you want to check out these classes, go to this website, www.WaterBikingStudio.com! Possibly another trend, but definitely one that I want to try!

And if you spend long hours at your desk or have to take long flights, there is another new device called the Flyte Bike (www.flytebike.com), a portable pedaling device you can take anywhere. It will fit in any carry on and is very light to pack. If you are on a plane, it fits right under the seat in front of you. With the risk of developing clots while traveling long distances, this is a great tool! On my last flight, the flight attendants were always going up and down the aisles with their big carts with food and drinks, and there was a lot of turbulence, so we had to be seated for most of the six-hour flight. I was wishing I had one of these, especially when I finally stood up—ouch! Flyte Bike's motto is: "Don't just sit there! Pedal!"

Swimming and Group Classes

Swimming is a zero-impact activity. There is no pounding on the joints, and you can get a great cardiovascular workout that works the whole body. Swimming is great for most people, including high-level athletes and also those who are overweight, have arthritis, or impact-related injuries. Plus, if you have extra body fat, it will actually help you stay closer to the surface of the water since fat floats. Swimming, however, does require technique. Make sure you are comfortable with the basic swim strokes before you swim for fitness. If you are rusty, take a class.

If you really don't like to swim or don't know how, you can still get results from working out in the water. Running in the water is great exercise, and there are some training centers that actually have treadmills in the water. Also, if you love the water, music, and want a great workout, try a water aerobics class. Even though working out in the water is a nonimpact activity, the resistance of the water while moving can get you into shape very quickly.

Jump Rope and Rebounding

If you like to jump, how about trying a jump rope program or a rebounder? In order to jump rope, you should have healthy knees and also a good rope. There are some that are weighted, which makes the workout even harder. Put on some music and get going. Believe it or not, 5 minutes feels like 30 minutes when you are jumping rope, so start in small increments.

A better alternative for most seniors is the rebounder which is a small trampoline you can jump and run on without the shock to your knees, hips, and back. Also, rebounding is great for the *lymphatic system* which helps rid the body of toxins and also fight infections. Kids love to jump on trampolines just for fun! My dad, who is ninety-three years young, jumps on one every day and he is in awesome shape. He is having fun doing an exercise he loves! If you want to feel like a kid again, get a rebounder, put on some music, and start jumping!

Cardiovascular Equipment

You can find a wide assortment of cardiovascular training machines in any gym. With the advancement of technology, these machines can give you immediate feedback on heart rates, distance covered, calories burned, and time elapsed. You can also watch your favorite program or read a magazine or do a crossword puzzle while working out. Instead of vegging on a couch watching a program, why not watch it while you are working out? It makes it so much more fun, and you get to kill two birds with one stone.

Some of the more popular machines include rowing machines, treadmills, steppers, ellipticals, and cycles. It's fun to try them all and see which ones you like the best. Some people purchase these for their own home use so they don't have to go to the gym.

If you are like me and tend to get bored easily, you can choose two or three of these machines and combine then into one workout. For example, work out for 10 minutes on a treadmill, and then go 10 minutes on a bike, and then 10 minutes on a rowing machine. That's 30 minutes and the time flies by!

Dance, Dance, Dance!

I once had a student in my weight-training class who was there to lose weight but wasn't getting the results she wanted. I told her that she needed to add cardiovascular exercise to her resistance workout, but she said she didn't like to move much. She just liked to lift weights.

After giving her a list of choices and class examples, I finally asked if she liked to dance, and she said that she loved dancing! I had a friend who owned a club and so I told her to go to the club twice a week and dance for a full set of music without stopping. She did it, had a great time, and the weight started to come off. Plus, she met her future husband there!

So, do you want to dance? There are so many different types of dancing, and most of the time, you don't even need a partner! One of our more popular classes at the college is Line Dancing, and it is a great cardio workout and the students love it! Also, Zumba is really popular.

Not into learning routines? Try Pulse, a new workout that focuses on moving to the beat and freestyle moves. If you are the shy type, put on some music at home and dance as if no one is watching. If you want to try something new, effective, and fun, put on those dancing shoes!

Play a Sport

You probably played a sport when you were younger and enjoyed it and also got fit doing it. Well, it's never too late to get back into the game! You can take sports classes at most colleges and recreation centers. Some of our most popular classes at the college are soccer, volleyball, softball, basketball, tennis, and sand volleyball. Besides learning the techniques of the sport, you will get opportunities to test out your skills by participating in competitions.

If you want to really get back into the game, join a team or a league! Recreation programs and clubs always have teams looking for participants. Not only will you be trying to win, you will also be working on your social skills because you will have to get along with your teammates—something a lot of people can't seem to do in the real world. So consider joining a team. You might be surprised how quickly you can adapt and how much fun it will be to get in shape and also work toward a team goal.

One of the new sports that's gaining a lot of popularity is pickleball (www.pickleball.com). It is a paddle sport that combines elements of badminton, tennis, and ping-pong and was created for all ages and skill levels. The game is easy to learn and the rules are simple, but I know many people who are really competitive. You can play it either indoors or outdoors and as singles or doubles. If you are game, why not try a new sport?

Workout Videos and Online Workouts

There are so many amazing workout videos and online programs; it's enough to make your head spin. These are great for traveling! You can have them on your computer, iPAD, or phone. I subscribe to a service that is only $9.95 a month, and I get new workouts delivered every week. Check out www.fitfusion.com if interested.

Some of the videos I have on hand are Insanity (A HIIT workout), the Ultimate Yogi (power yoga), and the Navy Seal Training Camp Video Series (boot camp). I know, these are intense but I find them to also be entertaining and fun.

Therefore, if you want to work out on your own, start getting your own library together. Then, when you are feeling lazy and need to get off the couch and move, pop one of these into your player and get moving.

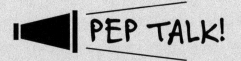

Wouldn't it be nice if when you went to a restaurant, you could have a small sample of anything you wanted on the menu before you ordered? Well, finding your own workouts are kind of like that. Get out and explore! Find the workouts that you not only enjoy but you also can fit into your schedule. And choose more than one! Not only will this eliminate boredom but they will also give you faster results.

I hope you'll get out and try some of the workouts mentioned in this chapter!

CHAPTER 5

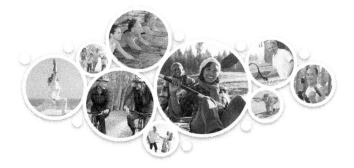

Resistance Training for Muscle Strength and Endurance

No fitness program is complete without *resistance training*. Resistance training is any exercise that causes the muscles to contract against an external resistance. Even though cardiovascular endurance is sometimes considered the most important fitness component, our muscles need to be conditioned in order for us to be able to do our daily activities. Having a strong heart and a lean body are great, but our muscles are what move us around in life, and if we don't use them and train them against resistance, we risk losing them.

Also, consider this: If you had a blob of clay, you could sculpt it into whatever shape you wanted to. Well, consider that your body is a blob of clay. With most cardiovascular activities, that blob will become a smaller blob but won't have any shape. With resistance training, once you learn the basics, you can sculpt your own body because you can target muscles. Isn't that cool?

Here are some of the benefits of resistance training:

- Increases muscle strength, endurance, and power
- Improves sports performance
- Challenges a person
- Increases muscle mass
- Increases basal metabolic rate (BMR) so a person burns more calories at rest
- Relieves stress and anxiety
- Improves posture
- Offsets muscle imbalances
- Prevents the loss of muscle mass that occurs with aging
- Encourages people to go to "failure." (*Failure* in weight lifting means doing a particular exercise until you can no longer lift with good form. *Failure* in resistance training is considered success! Individuals experience failure with their self-esteem intact.)
- Heightens *kinesthetic awareness* (Internal awareness of the body) and sensitivity to our body's needs. You will definitely be able to feel muscles you never even knew you had.
- Reduces the risk of falls.
- Everyday physical activities become easier.
- Resistance exercises burn calories both during the exercise period and also after the workout.

Most men are very familiar with the benefits of weight training. They know that resistance training increases strength, builds quality muscle, and improves performance in whatever physical activities they are involved in. But many women tend to shy away from weight training because they fear that they will start to look masculine or gain weight. Trust me; women will never get huge muscles from resistance training unless they take anabolic steroids and train excessively.

Here are some weight-training benefits specific to women:

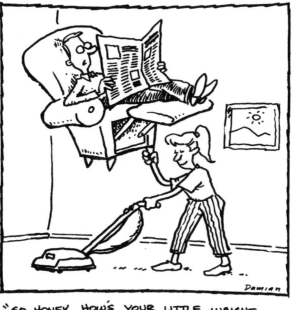

"SO HONEY, HOW'S YOUR LITTLE WEIGHT TRAINING CLASS GOING?"

- Resistance training provides shapely, firm muscles that cannot be obtained by dieting or aerobic exercise alone.
- Because women have low levels of the male hormone testosterone, they DO NOT get excessively large muscles from weight training. The muscles respond by increasing in density. Instead of getting big muscles, women tend to lose inches, slim down, get a more defined body, and develop strength.

- Muscles weigh more than fat. This might cause some women concern because they tend to get upset when they see the weight on the scale either stay the same or increase, especially if they have been working hard. If a woman is doing resistance training, she needs to use other methods to track progress, like doing measurements or a body composition test.
- The more muscle mass you have, the more you can eat. I always ask my female students if they have boyfriends or brothers who can eat anything and not put on weight, and most of them raise their hands. I tell them not to get mad. Get even! They can get that fast metabolism too by putting on more muscle!
- Weight-training increases self-esteem and may also relieve PMS and menopausal symptoms.

One of the best things about resistance training is that it doesn't take a lot of time to see results. All of the major muscle groups can be exercised in as little as 15 to 20 minutes, and you don't need to train more than twice a week unless you want to.

Before we start talking about different ways to use resistance training, first there are a few basic terms I'd like to introduce that make up the language of resistance training:

Hypertrophy: The enlargement of a muscle.

Atrophy: The shrinking of a muscle.

1RM: This is short for "one repetition max," which means the maximum amount of weight you can lift in one attempt. This is an indicator of muscle strength.

Momentary Muscle Failure: Exercising to the point where a muscle can no longer perform a contraction.

Rep: Short for repetition. One performance of an exercise.

Set: A group of repetitions followed by rest.

Individual Differences (*Bio-individuality*)

When it comes to individual differences, or what I like to call *Bio-individuality*, there is good news and bad news. The good news is that anyone can benefit from a resistance training program. The bad news is that it is easier for some and harder for others, and some people will have tremendous gains while others will have moderate gains. Some of the differences that influence how much you will benefit from resistance training include body type, muscle fiber-type distribution, level of fitness, gender, age, diet, and lifestyle.

Body Types

These are usually categorized according to the relative amounts of fat and muscle. Genetic predispositions play a role in determining body type, and you can only work with what you have. However, anyone can improve his or her body type through resistance training. There are three general categories of body types:

1. *Endomorph*: A person with this body type tends to have more body fat than average and less muscle mass.
2. *Ectomorph*: A person with this body type tends to have a lower-than-average amount of both muscle mass and body fat.
3. *Mesomorph*: This person has a higher amount of muscle mass than average and a lower-than-average amount of body fat.

Many people are a combination; for example, a person who has a large amount of both muscle mass and fat is a mesomorphic-endomorph. As we know, we cannot change our height or bone structure, but we can change the amount of fat on our bodies, and with a lot of hard work, the size and shape of our muscles.

And believe it or not, burning fat is much easier than building muscle.

If you have an endomorph body type, then it makes sense to do activities that are both aerobic and fat burning and also activities that develop muscle mass. Otherwise, you could end up with toned muscle mass underneath a thick layer of fat.

If you are have an ectomorph body type, obviously burning fat is not a priority whereas putting on muscle mass would be more of a primary goal.

A mesomorph usually has more than an average amount of muscle to begin with, so hypertrophy (increase in muscle size) and strength gains usually come quicker and are more noticeable.

Remember, you can't trade your body in for a new one, but you can do a major reconstruction job on the one that you have. It takes knowledge, motivation, and of course, action.

Muscle Fiber Types

A muscle cell is called a *fiber*, and there are basically two muscle fiber types: *slow twitch* and *fast twitch*. Each of these fiber types has unique characteristics. The *slow-twitch fibers* usually contract slowly, are thinner, have a high-aerobic capacity and therefore resist fatigue. The *fast-twitch fibers* contract fast, are thick, and fatigue rapidly.

The relative distribution of these fiber types is genetically determined. A world-class sprinter or power lifter would probably have a higher percentage of fast-twitch muscle fibers than a world-class endurance athlete, who would most likely have a higher percentage of slow-twitch muscle fibers. Many people have a 50/50 distribution, but others have more of one kind and less of the other.

You cannot change a slow-twitch muscle fiber into a fast-twitch muscle fiber. For this reason, people with a high percentage of slow-twitch muscle fibers have more of a challenge getting their muscles larger if that is what they desire. This is just another reason why people might respond differently to the same resistance-training program.

Level of Fitness

Here is some good news if you are out of shape. You'll improve faster than a person who is fit, the reason being that a person who is out of shape has a lot further to go and therefore notices changes sooner. A fit person's progress usually will be slower since he or she is already fit, and sometimes a fit person has to work hard just to maintain a high level of fitness.

Gender

Men are born with more muscle fibers than women. Also during puberty, their bodies start to secrete testosterone, which among other things, makes their muscles larger. For these two reasons, men usually show increases in strength along with muscle size. You can usually tell if a man is strong by looking at the size of his muscles.

Women, on the other hand, are born with less muscle fibers, and even though they do have some testosterone in their bodies, it is usually not enough to promote large musculature. When women get strong, their muscles get denser, not necessarily bigger. The only exception would be if a woman has a large amount of fast-twitch muscle fibers in a particular muscle group. However, since women don't normally have high levels of testosterone, it would be difficult to achieve the *hypertrophy* that men can develop with the same percentage of fast-twitch fibers.

Age

"Use it or lose it." We have all heard this before, and it applies directly to muscle mass and aging. As we get older, if we do not exercise, we tend to lose between one-quarter and one-half pound of muscle a year—more if we diet excessively. Muscle mass tends to peak in the early twenties and declines after age forty. This muscle loss is one reason why people become frail as they get older and also tend to get fatter.

By the age of sixty-five, muscle mass and strength decline by about 20 percent. People assume that we get fat and frail because of age, *but the truth is that we age because we get fat and frail.* What is so great about resistance training is that you are never too old to get results. You can reverse this decline and put muscle back on no matter how old you are.

Nutrition

You could have the greatest resistance program on the planet, but if you don't have a healthy diet, you might as well do nothing. Muscles need nutrients for both exercise and muscle repair. If you don't eat enough nutrients, your energy levels will be too low to lift anything, and the muscles will start to tear down instead of rebuild. Fatigue and injuries are common problems for people who lift weights but neglect proper nutrition. (See chapter 8.)

Lifestyle

How you live your life outside the weight room or gym can affect the results from your resistance program. If you smoke, drink, use recreational drugs, have unmanaged stress, or do not get enough rest, you run the risk of negating all the hard work you put into your resistance workout.

Safety Guidelines and General Lifting Techniques

Before you start a resistance-training program, it is important to know proper technique and safety guidelines. If you are a beginner, I would suggest you hire a trainer or take a class to make sure you don't get injured.

1. Breathe properly when working with resistance. Exhale on exertion and inhale during relaxation. Never hold your breath while training with weights.
2. Move only the parts of the body that are supposed to be moving in the exercise. Keep the rest of the body stabilized.
3. Use a full range of motion on all lifts.
4. Take 2 seconds to lift a weight and 4 seconds to lower it. Another rep speed is to use a 10-second count: Use 4 seconds to life the weight, hold it for 2, and then lower for 4 seconds. The slower rep speed actually stimulates more muscle fibers.
5. Rest approximately 60 seconds between each set.
6. Warm up the muscles before you lift any weights. Or you can warm up with an extremely light weight.
7. Cool down and stretch when you are done.
8. Ask for help if you need it. This is especially important for barbell exercises.
9. A muscle requires at least two days of rest to recover and adapt before it should be exercised again, especially if you went to failure during your sets.

10. Exercise the larger muscle groups first and the smaller ones last.
11. Listen to your body. If you become very sore or experience acute or chronic pain, this is not normal or desirable.
12. Never sacrifice form to add more weight.
13. When lifting a weight off the floor, keep it close to your body. Keep your back straight, your head up, and lift with your legs.

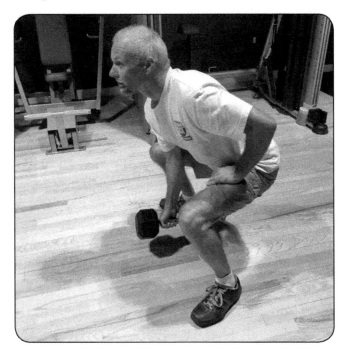

Muscle Balancing

Most of the muscles in the body work in pairs. This is important to remember when designing a resistance workout so the muscle groups don't become unbalanced. We see a lot of people in the gym just work the muscle groups that they want; for example, just working the biceps and not the triceps, or the chest and not the back.

If the muscle groups are out of balance, injuries can occur, especially dislocations or postural defects. For example, let's say that a person does a lot of exercises for the chest muscles, but doesn't work the upper back muscles. With the chest muscles being very strong and the back muscles weak, this could cause an abnormal forward curvature of the upper spine.

Let's Get Out the Clay!

Picture your body as though it were a blob of clay. Now, with the imagination of a sculptor, design the shape of the body you desire. Do you want a fuller, more defined upper body? A smaller waist and hip measurement? Larger calves? Smaller, more toned thighs?

Muscle sculpting is an art, and by using resistance, you can shape your body any way you want. Just remember to keep individual differences in mind as these differences can affect the amount of time and the extent of the changes possible. You can change the shape, tone, and size of any muscle in your body. In order to do this, you must understand the difference between muscle-endurance and muscle-strength training. The amount of weight, repetitions, sets, and length of rest between sets are specific to the results you will get. A general rule is, if you want to build strength or get hypertrophy, use heavy resistance with less repetitions. To develop muscle tone, use less resistance and more repetitions.

Here are some examples of guidelines for lifting for strength, endurance and tone, or a combination of both strength and endurance. Obviously these can all be modified for each individual based on their fitness, age, limitations, and overall health.

STRENGTH	
Weight:	80-90% 1RM
Reps:	5-10
Sets:	3-6
Rest:	At least 1 minute between sets
ENDURANCE AND TONE	
Weight:	50-80% 1RM
Reps:	12-20
Sets:	2-4
Rest:	At least 30 seconds between sets
COMBINATION: STRENGTH AND ENDURANCE	
Weight:	70% 1RM
Reps:	8-12, or for people over 65, 10-15
Sets:	1-3
Rest:	60 seconds between sets

These are just examples, but I think you can see the basic differences. There is also an obvious overlap in resistance training. If a person decides to train for strength, or hypertrophy, muscle tone will probably also improve. Also, if a person decides to train for tone or endurance, some improvement may occur in strength and size.

The question is what do you want the MOST?

Remember, you are not shaping fat; you are shaping muscle. You do not burn fat from the area you are working. Unfortunately, fat usually comes off in the reverse order you put it on. First on—last off! That's why it is important to have a cardiovascular program to go along with resistance training.

Remember my student in the weight-training class from the last chapter? When she finally found an enjoyable cardiovascular activity, she really started to see results. And all she had to do was dance!

Resistance Machines versus Free Weights

I get this question all the time: What's better, free weights or resistance machines?

It depends on the individual. For beginners, I usually recommend that they start with the machines because of safety concerns.

The advantages of working out on the machines are that they require little skill, are usually safe, spotters are not necessary, and they provide more resistance than free weights. The disadvantages are they are expensive to buy, take up a lot of room, and the exercise variety is limited. You can only work the muscles in the range of motion that the machine allows.

With free weights (dumbbells and barbells), the advantages are they are cheap to buy and maintain, allow greater variety of exercises, and also allow the muscles to work in different ranges of motion. The disadvantages are that safety is a concern because the weights can be dropped and cause injury, and they also require more skill and technique, and some of the lifts require a spotter.

It really is up to you as to what you think will give you the best results and what you will enjoy doing. They both work, that's for sure!

Where to Begin?

The most common mistake for a beginner is overtraining. People tend to overestimate their starting strength and end up either injuring themselves or getting so sore that they never want to lift again. If this is your first time, start slow.

Most trainers and experts recommend in the early stages of a program the use of light resistance—60-70 percent of a max lift and a range of 8-12 reps or 10-15 reps for people over sixty-five years of age (50-60 percent of a max lift). It usually takes a while to find what weight you can comfortably lift in those ranges. A good rule of thumb is to go with a 5 on a scale of 1-10 of difficulty.

Eventually, as that weight starts to get easy, you can increase the weight or the reps, depending on your personal preference. Exercising one set of the major muscle groups twice a week is enough to stimulate results in a beginner. As you get stronger and more familiar with the lifts, more sets can be added.

Here is a sample weight-lifting program utilizing resistance machines.

BENCH PRESS   **SEATED ROW**

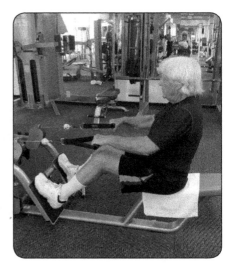

OVERHEAD PRESS

LAT PULLDOWN

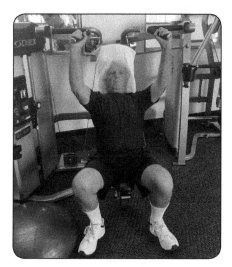

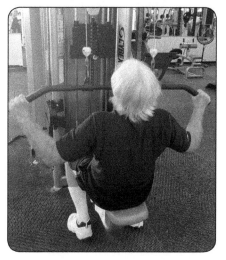

BICEP CURL

TRICEPS EXTENSION

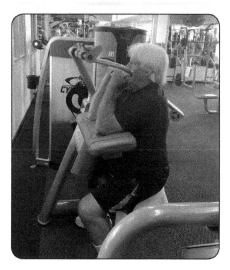

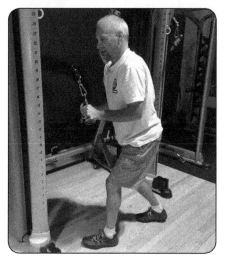

LEG PRESS

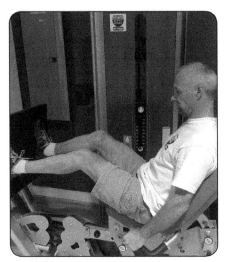

HAMSTRING CURL

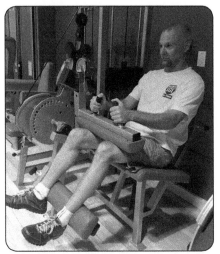

ABDOMINAL CURL

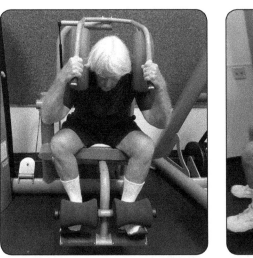

LOW BACK PRESS

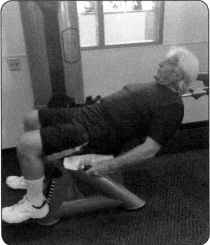

You might notice that these are most of the major muscle groups, and the workout is balanced for the muscles on both sides of the joints.

How to Get the Most Out of Your Resistance-Training Program

The following guidelines will help you fine-tune your program to meet your goals. There are many resistance programs available, and the next sections will show you how to get creative!

- Use specificity. Train the way you want your body to change. If you want muscle tone, use light weights and do a lot of reps. If you want to build muscle, increase the weight and decrease the number of reps. If you are weight training for a sport, find out the physical demands of the sport and apply them to your program.
- Work on your weaknesses. If you have weak legs, they should be more of a priority than a stronger upper body.
- Eat a well-rounded, sensible diet. Make sure you have enough energy to fuel a workout by eating complex carbohydrates at least two hours before a resistance workout. After your workout, make sure you eat some protein to help rebuild muscle, especially if you are training for strength.
- Establish a year-round program. Have several types of resistance programs available for variety and to push through plateaus.
- Make sure you adapt to a workout before you "overload." In other words, get in shape gradually. Doing too much too soon will only cause soreness and risk injury.
- Do not do resistance training if you are injured. Give the injury time to heal.
- Use "periodization" to vary the volume and intensity of your workouts. Have some hard days followed by easy days.

- Work out with a partner at times. This buddy system not only helps with motivation, but also helps to ensure safety, especially when lifting heavy free weights.
- Increase the reps before you increase the resistance. This gives your body time to adjust to the demands of the exercise.
- Record your exercises, reps, and sets on a workout chart or card. Also, if you have any questions about any exercise or your program, make sure to ask a trainer or a teacher.

Are You Ready to Get Creative with Resistance?

Resistance training has become both an art and a science. There are many workout variations and systems available, and some of them are really fun!

Most people do what is called *straight sets* or *fixed loads*. In other words, the resistance reps and sets remain the same for a training session; for example, doing a leg press exercise using 160 pounds, 10 reps, 3 sets. All three sets are the SAME. That's good enough to get results, but after a while, it can get BORING!

The following is an example of *varied sets*. As you can see, the weight and reps change with each set.

Set 1:	160 pounds	10 reps
Set 2:	150 pounds	12 reps
Set 3:	140 pounds	15 reps

You get the idea. Each set is different depending on the results you want to achieve.

You could also add more sets and make some *ascending(moving up in resistance or reps)* and others *descending (moving down in resistance or reps)* . I like the following example for a bench press because you get the best of both:

Set 1:	60 pounds	12 reps
Set 2:	80 pounds	8 reps
Set 3:	100 pounds	5 reps
Set 4:	80 pounds	8 reps
Set 5:	60 pounds	12 reps

Now that is a workout that is also effective!

Another fun workout is to add *supersets*. This is when you perform two different exercise sets and then rest. Usually *antagonistic pairs* (muscles on both sides of a joint) are exercised in this manner. An example would be to do a leg extension set followed immediately by a leg curl set and then resting before doing it again.

Also, people love to do *circuits*. This entails a series of exercise sets followed by a rest. Participants move from one exercise to the next and sometimes even do a cardio exercise in between, such as jumping jacks or rope jumping or running on the treadmill. Really, the combinations are endless. Circuits are both fun and produce great results because everyone is exercising and moving from station to station, and usually there is some great music to motivate people to move.

There is no reason to ever get bored doing resistance training! There are also group classes that do resistance training, and my two favorites are *body pump* and *suspension training*. Body pump is high-rep training, and when I say high, I mean high! Like over 60 reps in one set! There is a warm-up followed by a squat set, then a rest, then a chest set, rest, then back, rest, then biceps, rest, triceps, rest, shoulders, rest, abs, and then a final stretch. It is intense! Again, not much rest in between, usually only a minute. Suspension training utilizes a TRX Suspension Trainer made up of straps that leverage gravity and use a person's body weight to get fit. You can do hundreds of exercises and either take a class, or buy a TRX Suspension Trainer to use at home.

A Warning: Drugs and Weight Lifting

Anabolic steroids are drugs that mimic testosterone. Some athletes and weight lifters take these drugs with the hope of increasing athletic performance and muscle mass.

Some men and women as they age may need to take testosterone if their levels are not in a normal, healthy range. These people should be tested and have the testosterone prescribed by their doctors.

However, taking anabolic steroids just to enhance weight training or athletic performance entails many risks. Long-term steroid use has led to many health problems including heart disease, liver cancer, psychiatric disorders, and even death.

Also, women who take these steroids to enhance muscle mass can expect to become more masculine resulting in deeper voices, growth of facial and chest hair, acne, and unnatural increases in muscle mass.

The bottom line in using these drugs is even if they do increase muscle mass and physical performance, the gains are usually small and not worth the health risks. Always check first with your doctor and have your blood levels tested before taking any of these drugs.

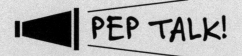

PEP TALK!

Are you more excited now about resistance training? Your muscles are counting on you to keep them healthy so you can get more out of life. Find a resistance training program that you enjoy and start it now! Remember to have fun with it and try something new every once in a while so you don't get bored or hit a plateau. Remember that in order for your body to be mobile for the rest of your life, you must have functional muscles. Use them! Don't lose them!

CHAPTER 6

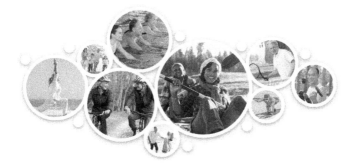

Flexibility and Yoga

Flexibility is just as important to your health as muscular strength and cardiovascular endurance. Being able to move your joints through their full range of motion without restriction or pain is something that people don't usually appreciate, that is, until they can no longer do it.

Most people work in flexibility along with their resistance and cardiovascular programs since they usually warm up and stretch before their workouts to prevent injury. However, stretching at the end of a workout is the best way to improve flexibility and also prevent soreness, especially after going to failure on lifting weights.

Even though flexibility varies from person to person and from joint to joint in the same person, it is something that we all need to work on. Just as we talked about "use it or lose it" in the last chapter on resistance training in reference to muscle mass, if we don't stretch, the tendons and ligaments and the actual muscle will all get shorter, and that's when it becomes hard to move. I don't know about you, but I want to be able to move restriction-free for the rest of my life.

Flexibility practices not only decrease risk of injury and increase the range of motion of joints, they are also a great tool to have for stress management. And there are so many ways to add stretching and a great flexibility practice into our daily lives.

Stretching Techniques

1. **Active Stretching**: When a muscle contracts, the opposing muscle stretches. Doing this slowly is a great way to warm up for any activity.

2. **Passive Stretching**: The stretching is facilitated by another person. Examples are partner stretching or being stretched out by a physical therapist or trainer.

3. **Static Stretching**: The muscle is held along its length for at least 10 seconds.

4. **Ballistic Stretching**: This is another name for bouncing while stretching. These stretches are usually not advised because the technique can injure soft tissue or contract a muscle into spasm if done too forcefully.

5. **PNF** (*proprioceptive neuromuscular facilitation*): This is very effective in getting results in range of motion. It is a contract-release technique where the muscle to be stretched is first contracted and held for 6-10 seconds, followed by a static stretch. This can be done alone or with a partner.

6. **Dynamic Stretching**: This one is done with slow, full body

motions. It is similar to active stretching but involves more muscle groups at the same time. It enhances the body's ability to safely elongate muscles. Yoga, and slow martial art practices such as tai chi and qi gong, are examples of dynamic stretching activities.

It doesn't really matter which technique is used—what does matter is that the muscles get stretched each and every day.

Stretching Tips

- Make sure you warm up the muscles before you statically stretch them. Muscles are like cold taffy when they are not warmed up. They can snap or tear if they are pulled too fast, too soon.
- For static stretching, hold the stretch, relax, and breathe deeply.
- NEVER stretch to the point of pain.
- For must stretches, keep the back in its neutral position.
- Do not compare yourself to others. Be content to work within your limits.
- Balance your stretches the same way you balance your resistance training. All muscles need to be stretched not just your favorites.
- Stretch only to light tension during a warm-up and to a great tension after cooling down.
- Close your eyes and tune into the muscle being statically stretched. Focus and become aware of muscle sensations and body alignment.
- Remember not to bounce while holding a static stretch.

Remember that most of your muscles work in pairs, so when you want to stretch a muscle, move the opposite way you would if you were doing a resistance exercise and hold the position. Most of us have our favorite stretches, and we need to honor our bodies when we stretch. "No pain, no gain" does *not* refer to flexibility training.

Yoga for Both Health and Fitness

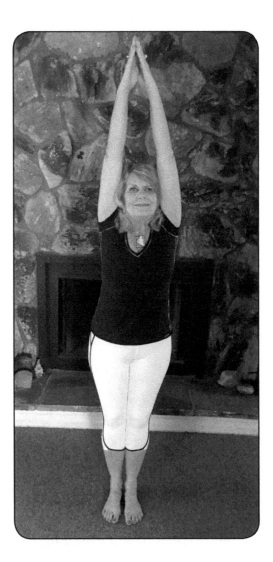

Most people think yoga is just about stretching, but it is so much more. It not only provides an amazing flexibility workout, it also can be both a cardiovascular and muscle fitness workout. Also, it has amazing benefits not only for the whole body but also the mind and spirit.

Yoga was not initially something in which I was even the slightest bit interested. As an athlete, coach, mother, and full-time teacher, when was there time to practice yoga, and what could it possibly offer someone like me? I had no desire to sit and contort my body into strange-looking positions.

However, one of my students in my health class asked me about the health benefits of yoga, and I really had no clue about how to answer him. Being a person who really wanted to know everything I could about improving heath especially since I taught contemporary health at the college I decided to do some research.

Coincidentally, a new yoga studio had just opened up in our town and was offering incentives to attract new members. Since the studio was within walking distance and the first class was free, I decided to try it. I felt a bit out of my comfort zone since I had absolutely no idea what to expect. My only clue was my husband's prized yoga book that showed an emaciated man on the cover wearing a turban with his legs looking like they were tied in knots above his head.

As I walked into the studio, I put my mat down at the back of the room and immediately noticed the feeling of serenity. Soft music was playing, people were doing some simple stretches, and the ceiling looked like puffy clouds.

A few minutes later, our instructor walked in. She was an extremely fit woman who looked like she could have been a high-level athlete. She introduced herself and explained to us "newbees" that we would move at a slow pace during class, listen to our bodies, not compete with anyone else, and rest whenever we wanted to in a position called a *child's pose.*

This was all new to me. In sports, I was always taught to push through pain, compete at any cost, and never rest unless I was hurt.

Even though I was in great shape at the time, I was surprised that I found myself struggling though the class. What a revelation to find my upper body was weaker than expected and that my shoulder and hip flexibility were sadly lacking. I felt like a foreigner in my own body. Out of the corner of my eye, I could see the other students moving effortlessly through the class as though it were a "moving meditation."

Every pose became a struggle for me as I attempted to execute it to perfection. Eventually, I had to listen to my body because it started to scream at me. Feeling defeated, I did rest in that strange child's pose that looked like a position assumed during an earthquake drill. My competitive nature was getting a well-deserved beating. At the end of the class, we were told to lie on our backs and rest in what was appropriately called *corpse pose.* With my body still shaking from the practice, I couldn't even hold that pose.

Finally, after several minutes, I stated to relax and my monkey mind finally let go of my body. I had been totally defeated by the yoga practice, and as a teacher I would have assigned myself an *F* for execution. But for the first time, I didn't care that I was terrible at yoga. I just wanted more.

So here I am seventeen years later as a certified yoga instructor with over 1,000 hours of training. While sports are still an important part of my life, yoga taught me to accept and work with my limitations and let go of expectations. Yoga is indeed a journey into self-discovery and a pathway to a healthy, productive life. And there are so many types of yoga out there! Yoga is indeed for everyone and there is no age limit!

The Health and Fitness Benefits of Yoga

For centuries, yoga's main goal has been to integrate the mind, body, and spirit. However, when we examine the definitions of *health* and *fitness*, it appears yoga is also a personalized path to attain ultimate health and fitness in today's busy, technology-filled, hurried world.

The World Health Organization defined *health* as "a state of complete, physical, mental, and social well-being, not merely the absence of disease and infirmity." Since that time, more dimensions have been added including emotional and spiritual well-being.

Doctors are responsible for our disease management, not our overall health. *Wellness* is our own movement toward optimal health, and having a consistent yoga practice is one way to achieve that because it addresses all of the dimensions, not just one.

Some of the physical benefits of practicing yoga include the following:

- Relieves arthritis
- Improves digestion
- Reduces risk of injuries
- Improves posture and spinal alignment
- Increases energy levels
- Increases lung capacity
- Promotes healing
- Boosts the immune system
- Relieves insomnia
- Promotes healthy skin

When it comes to mental and emotional health, yoga has exhibited success in improving these components because it enables the person to use an inner focus of control instead of relying on outside influences. Specific areas of improvement include the following:

- Lowers tension and anxiety
- Brings major stress relief
- Calms the chatter in the mind (monkey mind)
- Enhances awareness
- Allows present moment living (mindfulness)
- Improves concentration
- Enhances kinesthetic awareness
- Improves mood
- Alleviates depression
- Helps boost performance on cognitive tasks and improves memory

Spiritual health refers to a person's values and beliefs. Being healthy in this component does not require that a person practice a certain religion, or any religion for that matter. People often mistakenly believe that yoga is associated with a particular religion. While some people choose to add yoga to their religious beliefs, it is not necessary to do in order to get spiritual benefits. Yoga encourages self-exploration and how a person can help and serve others. Also, yoga improves our social health by helping us slow down and not be so reactive. One of my students said that her biggest benefit from yoga was that the people she works with don't call her a bitch anymore.

Some of the spiritual health benefits from yoga include the following:

- Promotes greater self-esteem and self- awareness
- Encourages us to live responsibly and consciously
- Opens us up to a higher perception of ourselves
- Helps us slow down and view situations differently and see the good in both ourselves and others

So yoga really does offer a holistic approach to improving our health. And even though yoga was not originally designed to improve fitness, modern forms of Hatha Yoga (the practice of physical yoga postures) can improve all of the fitness components, including cardiovascular fitness, muscle strength and endurance, flexibility, balance, and even with some of the more vigorous practices, body composition.

One of the greatest benefits of yoga is its ability to help manage stress. This is the main reason we added it into our curriculum at the college. The opportunity to take a break from life stressors and cell phones is a much needed time-out. When I tell my students they can't have their cell phones on their mats, some of them get upset, but I remind them that this is *their time* and they don't always have to be available for others 24/7. After a while, they really do appreciate the time away from the maddening crowds.

Also, the breath awareness and deep-breathing techniques practiced in yoga classes actually change the nervous system from a reactive fight or flight response, which gets us ready to either fight or run away from a stressor, to one of relaxation. The sympathetic nervous system that promotes the fight or flight stress response is activated in part by fast breathing and most people do tend to breathe very quickly. The parasympathetic nervous system that allows us to relax is activated by slow, controlled breathing. Yoga classes typically start with slow-breathing exercises, or *pranayama techniques,* that switch the nervous system from a reactive state to a relaxed state. AHHHH, so nice!

What Style of Yoga Is Best for You?

When a person decides to start a yoga practice, there are numerous choices. Yoga differs in forms, styles, and teachers so everyone is bound to find something that they enjoy while reaping the benefits. Know that variations of the same poses are common depending on the style practiced, along with different names for the same poses. What is important is to find one or more styles that work best for you and make yoga an integral part of your life.

The following styles of yoga can be found in most areas and many studios. While they are all different, the goals are the same—to integrate the mind, body, and spirit. While your goal might be to change your body composition or to become more flexible, be aware that you are getting other benefits as well. People who practice yoga typically notice that they are calmer, feel "lighter," and are better quipped at handling life's challenges. You will never get bored doing yoga because of the plethora of choices you have.

Level of Difficulty

Another element to consider when taking a yoga class is the level of difficulty. Most classes are level 1, 2, or 3, or a combination of them.

Level 1 is typically for people who are first discovering yoga or those who want a slower, easier practice.

Level 2 is intermediate and assumes that the participants have yoga experience and few physical limitations.

Level 3 is advanced, which means to be ready for anything.

Make certain you are matching the level of the class with your personal fitness and experience. Even if you are in great shape, it would be wise to start at the beginning level to learn the poses. You don't want to start at level 3 unless you want to be lost, dazed and confused, and really sore the next day.

The following styles of yoga are discussed in alphabetical order. If you want to check them out first online before you go to a live class, the websites are listed.

Ananda Yoga

Ananda Yoga is a classical approach that comes from the renowned yogi, Paramahansa Yogananda, author of *Autobiography of a Yogi.* Ananda Yoga rose from his teachings and was developed into a system of practice by his disciple, Swami Kriyananda. This classical approach includes postures, breathing and energy control techniques, meditation, and yoga philosophy. It is a gentle, inner-directed practice. Each pose is paired with an affirmation a person practices silently while in the *asana.* (yoga pose). Another unique feature of Ananda is the energizing exercises designed to increase focus and control the "life force."

Website: www.expandinglight.org

Anusara Yoga

Anusara Yoga is a modern style characterized by the "celebration of the heart." All levels and ages are welcome and honored for their uniqueness and talents. The class is based on the ancient Tantra philosophy that focuses on both alignment and awareness. Instructors are allowed to be creative; however, all classes start with an innovation and heart-oriented intention. John Friend is the creator of Anusara.

Website: www.anusarayoga.com

Ashtanga Yoga

Ashtanga Yoga is an athletic style based on Patanjali's eightfold path. Originated by Pattabi Jois, this style is one of the most athletic and challenging styles of Hatha Yoga. Ashtanga is designed to raise the body temperature and enhance strength, stamina, balance, and concentration. It includes six series that must be mastered in sequence before moving to the next level. In this class you will sweat, even though the room is not usually hot.

   Website: www.astanga.com

Bikram Yoga

Developed by Bikram Choudhury, this style of yoga consists of twenty-six postures performed twice in heated rooms usually above 105 degrees. This approach is vigorous and athletic but also therapeutic. The heat improves stretching and helps remove toxins from the body. All instructors follow the same dialogue and are not allowed to change the sequence of the poses. Just so you know, you cannot hide in these classes and must be able to see yourself in the mirror, whether you want to or not. Don't expect to be coddled. If you are doing the poses incorrectly, it will be noticed and you will be corrected. Also, you are expected to stay in the room for the whole time and the class is 90 minutes long, though some places just offer the first 60 minutes of the class. Make sure you not only bring your own mat, but also a towel and water. Plan to sweat like you never have before!

   Website: www.bikramyoga.com

Integral Yoga

This style of Yoga is an integration of Hatha Yoga with Karma and Bhakti Yoga. Hatha Yoga emphasizes physical discipline while

Karma Yoga emphasizes selfless service, and Bhakti Yoga emphasizes devotional practice. These classes are considered gentle and include guided relaxation, chanting, postures, breathing techniques, mantras, and meditation. In addition, they are peaceful and have a predictable routine. Swami Satchidananda, the founder of Integral Yoga, made his debut in 1969 at the Woodstock Festival where he taught thousands of participants to chant "om." This style is ideal for anyone seeking a more spiritual practice and those with physical challenges.

Websites: www.iyiny.org or www.yogaville.org

Iyengar Yoga

Created by BKS Iyengar, this is one of the most popular yoga styles in the West. Iyengar Yoga emphasizes precision in the poses and sometimes uses props such as belts, bolsters, and blocks. The poses are usually held longer than in most other styles, and the instructions are detailed. The emphasis of the practice is to heal the mind and the body. Instructors are trained to adjust students to attain proper alignment.

Website: www.bksiyengar.com

Kripalu Yoga

Kripalu Yoga is a journey into the self and also promotes the awakening of the "life force energy." This style is comparable with other styles and traditions of yoga practice and is considered "meditation in motion." Classes are variable depending on the teacher, but most include *asana (yoga poses)* , *pranayama (control of breathing)* meditation, and relaxation techniques. The focus is on awareness of the breath, body, and mind. Students are expected to honor the body and work according to their limits and strengths. This style is designed to immerse the student in self-inquiry and acceptance. The founder of Kripalu Yoga is Swami Kripalu, and the practice has been continued by Yogi Amrit Desai, one of his followers.

Website: www.kripalu.org

Kundalini Yoga

Kundalini Yoga is a strict spiritual discipline designed to release a form of energy residing in the base of the spine. The classes focus on repetitive movements, breathing exercises, and the repetition of mantras. The founder of this style is Yogi Bhajan, but several followers, such as Shakta Kaur Khalsa and Ravi Singh, have kept this energetic, unique and challenging style popular.

Website: www.kundaliniyoga.com

Power Vinyasa Yoga or Baptiste Yoga

Power Vinyasa Yoga is dynamic, rigorous, and sweaty. One of the main founders is Baron Baptiste who now calls his style *Baptiste Yoga*. He adapted this from several styles he was exposed to as a child in India, especially Ashtanga. There are several different variations of Power Vinyasa Yoga, or as it is sometimes called, *Power Yoga*. One thing is for sure—it is a workout! Baron's mantra is, "Don't Wait for It, Work for It." This style is taught in fitness facilities and is also common among athletes.

Power Yoga works on all the fitness components and does not require flexibility in order to participate, just a willingness to work hard. These classes include sun salutations which are intermediate and advanced poses that are held for long durations. This yoga is for anyone who really wants to work hard and push his or her limits. As

Baron used to tell his students (I was one), "The pose doesn't start until you want to come out of it." This style is definitely *not* for sissies.

Website: www.baptisteyoga.com

Viniyoga

Originally developed by Shri Krishnamachaarya and TKV Desikachar, this style of yoga emphasizes bringing out the best in each person. It requires an understanding of an individual's present condition, potential, and goals. Viniyoga serves to adapt the methods of yoga to the unique conditions, needs, and interests of each individual. As a result, students are given the tools to individualize the process of self-discovery. It is an unhurried, user-friendly approach to Yoga that incorporates sound, chanting, pranayama, asana, meditation, personal ritual, and the study of texts. Gary Kraftsow has expanded this style to allow accessibility to all searching for a yoga practice designed to fit their needs.

Website: www.viniyoga.com

Vinyasa Yoga

One of the most creative styles, *Vinyasa Yoga,* is a free-form style of yoga that is both fun and challenging. The nickname for these classes is *Flow.* The sequences are coordinated and connected with breathing, and certain sequences resemble dance forms. Shiva Rea is considered to be one of the base founders of this style, but others, mostly women, such as, Sean Corn, Ganga White, and Tara Stiles) have created their own variations. The classes can be challenging or meditative depending on the teacher, but the poses will be connected and flow with breathing. A moving practice for sure!

Websites: www.shivarea.com, www.seanecorn.com,
www.whitelotus.org

Yin Yoga

Yin Yoga combines yoga and meditation at the same time. Expect to hold some of the poses for five minutes. This style releases tensions, increases body awareness, improves flexibility, and enables participants to delve deeper into their individual spiritual nature.

Website: www.yinyoga.com

What's New with Yoga?

It seems that new trends are popping up every day when it comes to yoga practices. A lot of the new trends are actually fusion classes that combine yoga with other types of workouts, for example, weight training, martial arts, pilates, and dance. There are even some yoga classes that use elastic bands suspended from the air to help you go deeper in the poses (Aerial Yoga, www.aerialyoga.com).

Also, if you have trouble sleeping, try *Yoga Nidra* because it uses yoga to help with sleep patterns (www.dreamyogastudio.com). And if you want to have a lot of fun, why not try *Laughter Yoga* (www.laughteryoga.com)?

I do draw a line at some of these trends, though. The new *Goat Yoga* does not sound like fun to me. How can I do my yoga with a goat on my back? Also, *Beer Yoga* and *Pot Yoga* do not sound like classes I would try, and one I don't want to even think about is *Nude Yoga*.

But as you now know, there are many benefits of practicing yoga, so why not find a style you like and add it to your fitness program?

If you take a yoga class, common courtesy and sensitivity to others are necessities. The following list explains etiquette essentials for yoga classes. Everyone will benefit if these simple suggestions are honored:

1. **Get to class on time.** Arriving late to class is distracting and not appreciated. Even though arriving a few moments late is better than not practicing at all, you need to make sure you are not constantly tardy. This shows disrespect for the instructor and the other students. If you are late, come in quietly and go to the back of the room if possible.

2. **Turn off cell phones.** Remember that yoga is a time to move away from distractions and tune into the body. Turn off your phone, or even better yet, don't bring it to class. Nothing is more irritating than to hear someone's phone ring during class, even if it is a cute song. It will distract everyone, especially during the final relaxation or a guided meditation. Also, NO TEXTING during class.

3. **Remember that "Silence is Golden."** You should refrain from talking during a yoga practice and also from making noises, such as sighing or moaning. Please be considerate and save the socializing and noises for other occasions.

4. **Be fragrance-free.** Yoga classes are usually taught in small rooms, so if possible, shower before class and do not put on any fragrances. Many people are sensitive to strong scents. Also, if you smoke, refrain from doing so just before class.

5. **Be careful where you walk.** Yoga classes are usually done barefoot, so make sure you stay on your own mat, not only for your hygiene but also for the hygiene of other students. How would you like it if someone put his or her foot on your mat where you place your face during the child's pose?

6. **Don't compete or judge other students.** This is your time for you. It doesn't matter what anyone else does in class. Give everyone their own space and work on yourself.

7. **No kid zone.** Never bring small children to yoga unless you are attending a *Mommy and Me* class. Parents often atttend a yoga class to have some free time away from their kids, even if it's just an hour. Also, there are liability issues for the school or studio.

8. **Wear appropriate clothing.** The only occurrence more distracting than noises and scents is a major wardrobe malfunction. Remember that yoga puts your body into various positions, and some clothing will not keep certain body parts from being exposed. The clothing should be comfortable and allow you to move into poses without flashing everyone.

9. **Bring a towel.** Sweating is a sign that you are working hard and eliminating toxins. But don't drip sweat on anything except your own mat and towel. If you are leaving puddles on the floor, make sure you mop them up.

10. **Put your equipment away**. If you borrow a yoga mat, a strap, or a block, please put it away. Yoga instructors are not your maids.

Also, don't eat right before a yoga class. There are many compressions in most classes, and you don't want to feel uncomfortable while you are doing yoga. Also, remember to be patient with yourself. If you keep practicing, you will see improvement.

As a yoga instructor at a community college for the past seventeen years, I can honestly tell you that I have seen incredible transformations and results in my students each and every semester. So why not give it a try? If you don't want to go to a class, check out all the workouts online. You can set up your own area and enjoy all the benefits at home.

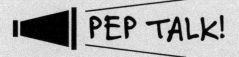

Remember that you are never too old to do yoga. Some of my students at the college have been in their seventies, and they never had a problem keeping up with the class. Also, there are always modifications, and if you go to a live class, just make sure you communicate with your instructor. He or she will offer some alternatives if needed. So if you haven't tried yoga yet, what are you waiting for? And if you try a class and don't like it, try another one. I promise that there is a yoga class that is perfect for you! You just have to be adventurous, get out there, and explore. And if you prefer to do yoga at home, there are several online workouts and DVD's. However, a live class is always more fun!

CHAPTER 7

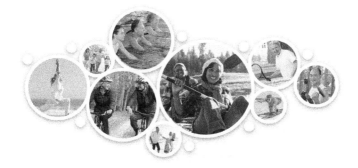

Avoid Injuries—Don't Get Hurt!

"No pain, no gain" does not apply to improving fitness or losing weight. Getting in shape is a slow, progressive process and for most people does not cause any problems. However, any form of exercise carries a potential for certain injuries; most of these stem from people trying to do too much too soon, or too much too often. Overuse is the primary cause of most exercise injuries. So make sure you tune in to what it feels like to have a good, safe workout and also what if feels like to overexert yourself.

Here are some body signs of a good workout:

- Breathing is controlled and comfortable.
- You feel like you can work at the same pace for an extended period of time (unless you are doing intervals).

- Shortly after the workout, you feel revitalized and full of energy.
- You have a good night's sleep after the workout and wake up refreshed.
- Any muscle soreness disappears when moving.

Here are some common signs of overexertion:

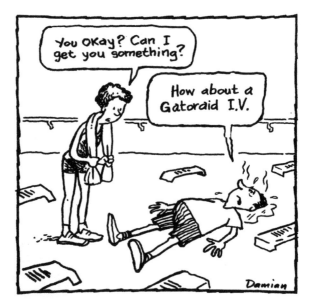

- Severe breathlessness
- Undue fatigue during exercise
- Dizziness, nausea, or feeling faint
- Severe muscle soreness
- Pain or tightness in the chest or extremely fast or irregular heartbeat (this requires a doctor's immediate attention)
- Inability to sleep at night
- Elevated resting heart rate

- Extreme hunger even after regular meals
- Extreme fatigue for the rest of the day following the workout
- Muscle soreness that does not go away

These symptoms do not mean that you should quit exercising. However, they do suggest you reduce the level of activity until you develop the capacity to handle the workload. Many people progress too fast for their bodies to catch up. Remember, it is important to start an exercise program slowly, and increases in frequency, duration, or intensity should only occur gradually after your body adapts to the exercise.

Acute versus Chronic Injuries

An *acute injury* is a sudden injury usually associated with a traumatic event, such as falling or getting hurt in a sport. Usually a sharp pain occurs and there is immediate swelling in the injured area. A *chronic injury* is usually caused by overuse and develops more slowly. Both injuries need our attention.

Common Exercise and Sports Injuries

The most common exercise and sports injuries include the following: muscle soreness and cramps, sprains, shin splints, stress fractures, side stitches, tendonitis, plantar fasciitis, and meniscus tears.

Muscle Soreness

This is the most common complaint of the beginning exerciser who insists on doing too much too soon. There are two different types of muscle soreness. The first type usually occurs during or immediately after an exercise session and disappears in three to four hours. The cause is an accumulation of lactic acid, a waste product resulting from working out without getting enough oxygen to the muscles.

The second type of soreness is called DOMS, which is an acronym for *delayed onset muscle soreness*, which is usually felt a day or two after the exercise period. DOMS is caused by minute tears in the muscle fibers and connective tissue. If you are just starting an exercise program, expect some soreness. Do not stop exercising because you are a little sore. Instead, make sure you stretch the areas affected and back off a little the next time you work that area.

Muscle Cramps

A *cramp* is a painful spasm in the muscles. Cramps can occur during an exercise session or even sometime after. The cause is usually dehydration and a possible electrolyte imbalance.

Make sure you drink water before, during, and after your exercise session. If you sweat a great deal during your exercise, the electrolytes can be replaced with a sports drink such as Gatorade or another one with less sugar. If you get a cramp, try to relax, slowly stretch the area, and make sure you hydrate by drinking a lot of water.

Sprains

A *sprain* is an injury to a ligament, which attaches one bone to another. Sprains occur when a joint is suddenly twisted or wrenched, causing the ligament to stretch or tear and often the blood vessels to rupture and bleed into the surrounding tissues. Symptoms of a sprain are swelling, discoloration, and tenderness. Normal motion will be limited by the swelling in the joints.

Sprains are classified by their severity. A *first-degree sprain* involves minimal stretching of the ligaments. A *second-degree sprain* involves tearing some of the ligament fibers, but the ligament is still intact. In a *third-degree sprain*, the ligament is completely torn off the bone.

Make sure you have good shoes that are designed for your activity and also offer support and traction. Also, avoid high-impact activities if you have arthritis or joint limitations.

If you do suffer a sprain, do not stand on it immediately as that can make it worse and take it longer to heal. The current treatment for most sprains is RICE—Rest, Ice, Elevation, and Compression although there is some new research suggesting that ice might not be the best treatment for everyone. And make sure you always see a doctor.

Shin Splints

The term *shin splints* refers to any pain or discomfort felt on the side of the lower leg in the region of the shin bone. If untreated, the condition can develop into stress fractures, which are more serious. Shin splints have many probable causes, including poor shoes, overtraining, exercising on hard surfaces, muscle fatigue, and insufficient warm-ups. To prevent shin splints, wear shoes with good shock-absorbing features and avoid weight-bearing, high-impact activities on hard surfaces. Also check out orthotics and insoles to help reduce the risk of shin splints and other foot problems. If you suspect that you might have shin splints, apply ice to the shins and reduce any activity that causes shock to the lower leg. If pain persists, activity should be limited and see a doctor if there is no improvement.

Stress Fractures

Stress fractures are small fractures that appear in a bone, which can cause the bone to break down gradually. There is usually a specific area of pain directly over the affected bone. The pain is sharp and radiating, and the area is usually tender to the touch. The most common sites of stress fractures are the feet and lower legs.

To prevent stress fractures, avoid repetitive activities on hard surfaces, wear proper shoes, orthotics or insoles, and increase exercise intensity gradually.

If a stress fracture is suspected, a doctor will most likely do an X-ray to determine how extensive the fracture is and how long it will take to heal.

Side Stitches

A *side stitch* feels like a sharp pain in the side of the rib cage. This is usually caused by a spasm of the diaphragm, which is usually caused by an insufficient supply of oxygen to the area due to decreased blood flow to the area. It most frequently occurs when a person has either recently had a meal or drinks a large amount of fluid right before a workout.

There is no simple treatment that works for everyone. Some people can continue to exercise while gently pressing their fingers in the painful area, while others have to stop and bend over or sit down and breathe deeply until the spasm subsides.

Tendonitis

Tendonitis is the chronic inflammation of a tendon. Tendons attach muscle to bones. Symptoms include swelling, pain, and some loss of function. Pain is usually the worst before any movement occurs. The pain will usually disappear after the warm-up and recurs when activity ceases. In advanced cases, the pain continues throughout the workout. The usual cause is overuse, and the common sites are the Achilles tendon and the patellar tendon crossing the kneecap. To prevent tendonitis, do not over train. Make sure you stretch before and after your workout, and if there is pain, applying ice to affected area may help relieve the discomfort.

Plantar Fasciitis

Plantar fasciitis is another chronic inflammation that affects the ligaments that fan out from the heel to the ball of the foot. It can lead to tears and bone spurs. Pain will be felt in the heel and under the arch. Usually, the affected area will ache in the morning, subside during the day, and get worse again at night. The usual cause is overuse and insufficient arch support.

To prevent plantar fasciitis, shoes must have adequate arch support, and high impact activities should be limited. Also, stretching the calf and Achilles tendon will help prevent this from occurring.

Meniscus Tears

A *meniscus tear* is a tear in the cartilage where the femur rests on the tibia. Pain may be felt inside the knee, and it may be difficult to flex and extend the knee, which may lock or give way. Any movement requiring a quick change of direction is difficult.

The usual cause is a sharp twisting action of the knee or forced bending or straightening of the knee. To prevent a meniscus tear, use body control and proper alignments, especially when performing squats and lunges. Treatment usually involves limiting any painful weight-bearing exercise, and sometimes surgery is required.

When Should You See a Doctor?

These are some surefire signs when you must see a doctor. Remember that exercise is supposed to help you get healthier and happier. If you have an injury, make sure you have it treated!

You should see a doctor if you have the following:

- An acute traumatic injury, such as an ankle sprain
- A chronic injury that recurs or suddenly worsens
- Specific point-tender pain, especially around a bone
- Any radiating pain that travels up and down a body part
- Fainting, disorientation, blurred vision, and nausea
- Swelling in any area for any reason
- Discoloration of the skin associated with an acute or chronic injury
- Impaired movement that limits the range of motion. If you are limping, see a medical professional!
- Weakness in a specific muscle or muscle group
- Trouble breathing
- Chest pain

Heat-Related Problems

Exercising in the heat presents problems for many people. Sweating is the body's main line of defense against overheating, but heat injuries can occur when the body is not able to dissipate heat appropriately. They are usually caused by a combination of a hot or humid environment, a high level of activity, and a lack of fluid replacement that causes dehydration.

You can avoid the following four heat-related conditions by drinking water before, during, and after the workout and also by reducing the intensity of the exercise whenever the environment is very hot and humid.

1. **Heat Syncope:** If you start to feel faint, stop exercising, get out of the sun, and drink cool water.

2. **Heat Cramps:** These can be in specific muscles, such as the *gastrocnemius* calf muscle, or can be multiple muscles cramping at the same time. For a specific muscle cramp, apply direct pressure to the muscle, stretch and massage the area, and ice. Also drink cool water.

3. **Heat Exhaustion:** The symptoms include nausea, headache, dizziness, weak and rapid pulse, profuse sweating, cold and clammy skin, shallow breathing, and possible loss of consciousness. To treat, elevate the feet and drink cool fluids and gently move or massage arms and legs. Move if possible to a well-ventilated area that is cool.

4. **Heat Stroke:** This condition is an extreme emergency. The symptoms include staggering, no perspiration, dry skin, being very hot with a temperature as high as 106 degrees, rapid and strong pulse, labored breathing. Call 911. Remove as much clothing as possible. Cool the body by using any means possible including ice, water, or a cool fan, and if it is someone else who is experiencing these symptoms, stay with the person until help arrives.

To eliminate the risk of heat injury, remember to drink water before, during, and after the workout and reduce the intensity of the workout when it is hot. You can also work out indoors in an air-conditioned facility. Also, do not wear any material that could interfere with the removal of heat from your body. If you ever start feeling nauseated, dizzy, or feel a headache coming on, stop exercising and start drinking water!

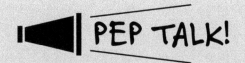

So, stay safe while exercising. Remember that the goal of a fitness program is to improve your health and vitality, and that exercise should be fun and make you feel great. It should never be viewed as punishment, cause pain or put you at risk for injury. So make your safety a priority and listen to your body not only when you are exercising, but also at rest. You only have one precious body. It's depending on you to take care of it!

CHAPTER 8

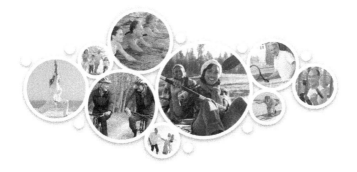

Fuel Your Workouts with the Proper Nutrition

Many people believe they can counteract poor eating habits with exercise. Even though a lot of people eat poorly and exercise, both good eating habits and exercise are important to achieve any health or performance goals.

As we get older nutrition becomes more important than ever. Most of the chronic diseases and disabilities associated with aging are related at least in part to our poor dietary habits.

Most athletes and fitness buffs know that if they eat poorly, they will not be able to live up to their potential, although there are some who exercise for hours a day but live on junk food or virtually no food at all. They might still be able to run, jump, and lift, but they are not really healthy and can end up getting sick or injured.

The bottom line is that you can't outrun your fork. Trust me; I have tried.

How we eat influences all aspects of life, including our work, energy levels, psychological status, and physical health. Unfortunately, most of us don't take our nutrition seriously and don't realize the power that food has to either help us—or hurt us.

It is ironic that Americans have the resources to eat better than people in most other countries in the world. However, most of our major killers are directly related to our nutritional habits. The excessive consumption of calories, fat, sugar, and also chemicals has been linked to most chronic diseases, including heart disease, cancer, diabetes, obesity, and also autoimmune disease. There is even evidence that poor nutrition can also put us at risk for certain mental disorders.

We all intuitively know how to eat well. However, in today's world, it's easier said than done. We live in a society where food manufacturers spend billions of dollars a year to advertise food, most of which is unhealthy.

In America, it is normal to eat foods that are unhealthy because they are fast (that is, can be prepared quickly), convenient, and taste good. The next time you take a drive in your car, notice how many fast-food restaurants you see. I'll bet you can't go two miles in a populated city without seeing at least one McDonald's. The next time you are in a grocery store, take a look at all the processed foods that are full of sugar and chemicals. Just read the labels. Also, when you watch television, how many ads are there for foods that you know are unhealthy? Some of the ads even use sex to sell their food products.

If you really want to see results from your fitness program and stay healthy and vibrant, you have to start taking your nutrition seriously.

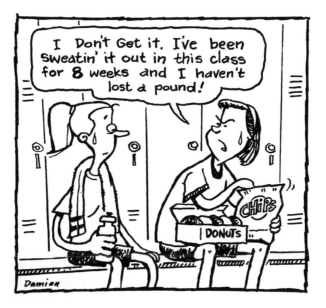

Nutrition 101

For starters, it helps to really understand how our bodies utilize food. Science classes teach us that our bodies are made up of cells that need both nutrients and oxygen to accomplish their various functions, and that they also need to have the toxins removed.

This sounds easy, but most of the food we eat doesn't have all the nutrients we need, especially the essential vitamins and minerals. What these foods do have is a lot of sugar and chemicals that the cells don't need at all. The extra sugar is stored as fat, and both sugar and chemicals play havoc with our hormones and which can result in chronic inflammation.

What is shocking is that average Americans take in over 90 percent of their calories by eating processed and fast foods. And then we wonder why we have so many chronic illnesses in our society. Some of these illnesses can be easily reversed if we just eat more nutritious foods and add more plant-based foods to our diets.

The Components of a Healthy Nutritional Plan

The following components are imperative to any healthy nutritional plan. They are moderation, balance, bio-individuality, and nutrient dense food. Restrictive dieting is not the answer to eating healthy. We should be able to enjoy food and not become obsessed with what we eat. Remember that we want food to fuel our lives; in other words, we want to eat to live, not live to eat. Big difference!

1. **Moderation:** This simply means not eating too much or too little. It seems that in our society, we follow the "all or none" law. We are either eating huge portions or dieting excessively.

2. **Balance:** Balance refers to the amount of calories taken into the body with the amount expended. You don't need to count calories to do this. If we just exercised for the same period of time that we spent eating, that would be a good start!

3. **Bio-individuality:** We are all different when it comes to the foods that we enjoy and also the ones that make us feel healthy. Don't go on a diet that proclaims it is designed for everyone. Learn to cultivate body wisdom by becoming aware of what foods make you feel healthy and perform at your best.

4. **Eat foods high in nutrient density:** This is easy to do if we just add more whole foods to our diet, such as fruits and vegetables. Mother Nature packages food perfectly

with both nutrients and fiber. For example, an apple is low in calories (about 60 in an average one), high in nutrients such as vitamin C, and high in fiber since it has pectin. Compare this with an apple pastry that has about 300 calories a serving, no fiber to make you feel full and packs a bunch of sugar and chemicals. See the difference?

So, what are the basic nutrients our cells need in order to function properly? See the following.

Basic Nutrients

The body needs more than fifty nutrients, which are divided into the following categories:

1. Macronutrients
   - Carbohydrates
   - Fats
   - Proteins
2. Micronutrients
   - Vitamins
   - Minerals
3. Fiber
4. Water

The *macronutrients* are large substances that provide calories. The *micronutrients* are smaller substances that are necessary for life processes but do not provide calories.

What Exactly Is a Calorie? (Kcal)

A *calorie* is a unit of measure that indicates the amount of energy obtained from a particular food. Calories are not the enemy. They fuel the body for all the body functions and activities. The problem is people consume more calories than the body can use and also eat foods that the body has trouble breaking down for fuel. Excess calories are stored in the body in the form of fat.

The nutrients that provide calories are: carbohydrates, fats, proteins, and alcohol. Any of these nutrients, especially processed foods and sugar, will be converted to fat in the liver and stored for "future use" in our adipose cells.

CALORIES PER GRAM

Carbohydrates:	4 calories per gram
Fats:	9 calories per gram
Proteins:	4 calories per gram
Alcohol:	7 calories per gram

Carbohydrates

Carbohydrates are the sugars, starches and fibers found in fruits, vegetables, grains and milk products. Most nutritional experts agree that more than half of your daily calories should come from carbohydrates because they are the body's main source of energy. All carbohydrates break down to glucose, which fuels the cells in the body for muscle contractions and basic body functions.

The problem these days is the way the glucose is delivered in our food. In order for the glucose to enter a cell, it has to be transported by insulin, which unlocks the cell in order for the glucose to enter.

Processed carbohydrates, (the bad carbs) consumed by most Americans, lack fiber and have a lot of sugar, which activate insulin to high amounts in short periods of time. It's too much too soon, and if a person continues to eat these foods, the insulin levels stay elevated and the body cells eventually become resistant and won't let the glucose into the cell. This is the perfect set-up for type 2 diabetes because the glucose continues to circulate in the bloodstream.

Also, the unused glucose eventually gets to the liver where it is converted to fat, and then the body ends up storing the glucose as fat. Sound familiar? And unfortunately, we can't reverse the process. Fat cannot be changed back to glucose.

Therefore, even though we need carbohydrates, we need to eat the foods that will deliver glucose to the cells slowly and not overload our bodies and cause the insulin to stay elevated. When you walk down the aisles in the supermarket, take a look at all the processed, refined foods we now have in our food supply. Is it any wonder we have problems with diabetes and obesity?

Another thing to remember is that if we want to lose weight and burn fat for fuel, once the fat has been stored, it can move out of the cells and go to the muscles to burn for fuel, but not if the insulin levels are still elevated. It is a one-way street! This might explain why some people who exercise or don't eat very many calories have trouble losing weight and even gain it easily.

So make the switch now and start adding more fruit and vegetables to your diet and start cutting back on processed foods. One of my friends is fifty years old and still plays competitive volleyball. He looks and plays like he is thirty. When I asked him what his secret was, he simply said that he never eats any food with a label. His fuel comes from whole foods, mostly fruits and vegetables. He considers a food label to be a warning label.

I know that eating like my friend would be hard for most people to do, but if we just cut down on these unhealthy foods and added more fruits and vegetables to our diets, these small changes could really add up to big results!

Also, there is always a controversy about organic foods and conventional foods. Organic foods have not been sprayed with pesticides and usually cost more. But if you are serious about being at your best, try to buy organic produce when you can, especially the foods that don't have thick skins, such as grapes, apples, and berries.

Remember that the chemicals in our food supply can wreak havoc in our bodies because our bodies see them as foreign substances. Therefore, these chemicals can activate our immune system, and if our immune system stays chronically elevated—just like with chronically elevated insulin levels—it can cause problems. Many of our chronic diseases are caused at least in part by chronic inflammation where the body starts to attack its own tissues.

So do yourself a favor—clean up your carbs!

Fats

Most people are so obsessed with their desire to get rid of body fat that they blame the fat itself. Fat is the most efficient way to store the energy that we have and is probably the reason why a lot of our ancestors survived during famines.

We also need fat to make hormones, help absorb certain vitamins, maintain healthy skin and hair, provide insulation, and stimulate brain health.

In order to be healthy, we need a certain amount of fat. But certain types of fat are healthier than others. Many fats come from animal sources and milk products, and others can also be found in plant sources, for example, avocados.

The healthy fats we need in our diets are the *omega 3s, medium-chain saturated fats*, and *monounsaturated fatty acids*.

We hear a lot these days about Omega 3s and how healthy they are to have in our diets. But what are they? The three types of fatty acids found in omega 3s are ALA (alpha-linolenic acid), EPA (eicosapentaenoic acid and DHA (docosahexaenoic acid). ALAs are commonly found in plant oils and both EPAs and DHAs are found in marine oils and fatty fish. They are all important for our metabolism, brain, and may help prevent heart disease and certain forms of cancer.

A while back, we demonized all saturated fats blaming them as a cause of heart disease. However, medium-chain saturated fats are smaller than the long-chain saturated fats and are easily digested and immediately converted to energy for both activities and body processes. One of the best sources of medium-chain fatty acids is coconut oil, which also contains lauric acid that has antiviral properties. No wonder people are now using coconut oil both to cook with and also on their skin!

Another healthy source of fats is *monounsaturated fats*, commonly called MUFAS. They can be found in olive oil, nuts, and also avocados. In terms of health benefits, they can increase resting energy expenditure, decrease anger and irritability, and also reduce levels of LDL, known as the bad cholesterol.

The most dangerous fats are the *trans fats*, and luckily, we are finally starting to take these out of our food supply. *Trans fats* are created when polyunsaturated oils are turned from liquid fats into solid fats by adding hydrogen through a process called *hydrogenation*. If a label has an ingredient that reads "hydrogenated vegetable oil" or "partially hydrated vegetable oil," then it contains trans fats, which increase the risk for heart disease and also increase the LDLs in the body.

Therefore, when it comes to fat, aim to make healthy choices to fuel your workouts and help prevent disease. Try adding healthy fish, like salmon, to your diet, along with nuts, olive oil, and coconut oil. Also try to avoid or cut down on red meat, which is very high in long-chain saturated fats, which, if eaten in high amounts, can put people at risk for inflammation and chronic diseases.

Most dieticians will recommend that our dietary intake should not be more that 30 percent in the form of fats, and no more than 10 percent should come from saturated fats. However, when we see how people typically eat, most Americans take in more than 40 percent of fats every day. We can thank most of the fast-food restaurants for that statistic. (I think they should change the name from fast-food restaurants to *fat-food restaurants*.)

In addition, restaurants are notorious for adding rich, fatty sauces to their foods and also serving huge portions. Check out the nutritional information online *before* you go to the restaurant. You might be shocked and surprised as to just how much fat is in their food and how many calories are in one entrée. For example, one of my favorite dishes at a popular restaurant had 2,400 calories with over 60 grams of fat. I never knew this until I checked it out. That's more calories than I should have in one day! And that didn't include the bread, the salad, the wine, or the cheesecake.☺ YIKES!

Protein

Protein is an essential nutrient needed by every cell in the body. Proteins make up the basic structure of all living cells and are essential for the formation and maintenance of all body cells. Protein also helps form antibodies that fight disease and hemoglobin that transports oxygen throughout the body. Protein is the most abundant substance found in the body other than water.

What is amazing is that adults do not need a lot of protein in the diet unless they are doing high-resistance training. Because muscles do break down in high-resistance training, they need protein in order to repair themselves and build new muscle.

Thus, our challenge is to get quality protein in our diets that have all the essential amino acids, which are the building blocks of protein. There are proteins in both animal and plant products. Animal products such as meat, milk, and eggs contain all the essential amino acids and are considered *complete proteins*. Plant sources of protein are beans, grains, nuts, seeds, and some vegetables also contain protein. Quinoa is an excellent source of protein, and it contains all the amino acids, however some of the other plant sources must be combined in order to get the desired amino acids.

Can people work out and be good at their sport and maintain their muscle mass if they are vegetarian? Of course! A gorilla eats plants. Does a gorilla have a lot of muscle? Absolutely! They just need to eat a lot of different types of vegetarian meals.

Protein supplements are very popular today, and many of them provide as much as 24 grams of protein per serving. I usually don't recommend these products unless people are on a resistance-training program. Excess protein in the diet overloads the kidneys and can cause health problems as a result.

The FDA recommends that people take in approximately 50 grams of protein a day based on a 2000- calorie diet. [1] Some people can eat up to 150 grams a day or more if they are physically active and some programs suggest that people who are trying to lose weight can also increase their protein intake because protein is filling and causes

---

1   healthyeating.sfgate.com/fda-daily-recommendations-protein-10249.html

people to eat less. However, if you have any kidney problems, do not go above 50 grams a day unless you check first with your doctor.

Vitamins and Minerals

Vitamins are organic (living) compounds required in small amounts for specific body functions. They don't supply calories; however, if you are deficient in certain vitamins, you may feel lethargic and fatigued. Vitamins help to convert food into energy and are also important for growth, maintenance, structure, and repair.

There are two main categories of vitamins. Water soluble vitamins are all the B vitamins and vitamin C and are not stored by the body. Fat soluble vitamins on the other hand are dissolved in fat can be stored by the body, and therefore we need to be careful that we don't take in too much. Vitamin D, K and E are fat soluble vitamins so high doses are potentially toxic and should be avoided.

Minerals are inorganic (non-living) substances that serve a variety of functions in the body. Without minerals, we would not be able to absorb some of the vitamins, so we need both. Some minerals we need in fairly large amounts and are referred to as *macro minerals* These include calcium, magnesium, phosphorus, potassium, chlorine, and sodium. We need other minerals in much smaller amounts; they are usually called *trace minerals. or micro minerals.* These include iodine, iron, manganese, selenium, zinc, chromium, cobalt, copper, and fluorine.

Do We Need to Take Vitamin and Mineral Supplements?

For some people the answer is no, and for others, a definite yes! When I have my college health students write down what they eat in a typical day, I wonder how some of them are still alive. Unfortunately, most of them eat snack foods, soft drinks, processed foods, and fast foods. Most of them don't eat any vegetables unless you count the lettuce and tomato on their hamburgers. SAD!

We can get all the vitamins and nutrients we need from eating natural whole foods; however, most Americans fail to get enough magnesium, vitamins A, B, C, D, and E, zinc, and many other trace minerals. The average woman does not get enough calcium and iron. So most people do need to take supplements.

It's not very often that I meet someone who doesn't need them. However, just a multivitamin and mineral supplement should work for most people. Also, some people have trouble absorbing nutrients from pills or have trouble swallowing them, so taking vitamins and minerals in liquid form is recommended for those people.

However, it is not advisable for people to take megavitamins that sometimes contain more than ten times the Recommended Daily Allowance. Only if a doctor has tested your blood and found a vitamin or mineral in very low amounts should you supplement that individual vitamin. For example, many people are taking vitamin D supplements because they don't get enough in their diets or do not get enough sun exposure.

Fiber

I have a good story on fiber. A while back I attended a workshop on nutrition, and the topic was how important fiber is in our diets and what can happen if we don't get enough. The presenter showed a video of two medical examiners performing an autopsy to determine the cause of death of a patient. When they opened up his intestines, they found over 80 pounds of fecal material that were stuck in the colon. Our presenter said that he had a condition called FOS.

When we asked what that meant, he said that FOS was an acronym for Full of _hit. And he added that most Americans have this condition because of the lack of fiber in the diet. YIKES!

Wow! I never forgot that one, and I always share it with my health students. So why do we need fiber again? To move the wastes out of the body. Fiber also helps us feel full so we don't eat too many calories.

Most processed foods have hardly any fiber, whereas whole fruits, vegetables, seeds, whole grains, and nuts have a ton. We need at least 25-30 grams of fiber a day to keep our digestive system healthy. The average American only gets between 10 to 15 grams a day. The next time you eat a processed food, check to see how many grams of fiber it contains. I'll bet it's less than 3 grams.

So do yourself a big favor. Start eating more foods with fiber.

Water

Water is the most important nutrient of all. More than 60 percent of your body is water, and on average, we lose about ten cups of water a day through sweating, urination, and breathing. This loss must be replaced. People can go without food for months and live, but without water, death can occur within days. Our body cannot store excess water the way it stores excess fuel.

Even though water does not contain any calories (unless it's been flavored), it is necessary for energy production, temperature control, elimination, and creating an environment in which all metabolic processes occur. Every cell in the body depends on water to carry out its essential activities. Water also maintains blood volume and blood pressure and carries nutrients and oxygen to muscles and organs. Water is vital for weight loss since it enables fat metabolism.

Water is present is some foods, but nutritional experts still recommend that we drink a minimum of six to eight glasses daily, although some people might need more or less depending on activity levels. Remember that thirst is not an accurate indicator of the body's need for water, especially when exercising. That's why you should always drink water about 30 minutes before exercising, and also drink water if you can during your exercise period and after exercising, too. If you weigh yourself right after a workout and find that you lost weight, don't get too happy. That weight loss is water loss and it must be replaced. For every pound that you lost, drink eight ounces of water.

How can you tell if you need to drink more water? One way is to take a look at your urine. If it is clear or a pale yellow, you are drinking enough. But if it is a dark color, you probably need to start drinking more. Also people who drink enough water usually have soft stools as compared to people who have hard bowel movements or constipation. These are just easy signs to be aware of in terms of keeping well-hydrated.

I always recommend that people carry water with them. Sometimes, when we think we are hungry, instead we are thirsty. When a person loses approximately 5 percent of the body's water, symptoms will start to occur, such as a weak and rapid pulse, headache, dizziness, and general weakness.

So the number one nutrient you need to get more of is most likely water! When I tell my students that most of them are not getting enough water, I usually have a female student tell me that she can't drink more water because she retains water. I respond by telling her that the best thing she can do is to drink more water and cut out the diet drinks. It's the sodium in your system that retains water. Sodium holds up to fifty times its own weight in water and causes bloating and temporary weight gain. Therefore, drinking more water will flush out the excess sodium in the system and release the excess water. I had one student cut out all diet drinks and she lost 5 pounds in one week. Obviously, it wasn't fat; it was retained water!

What Should You Eat before a Workout?

My fitness students always ask what they should eat before and after class. Remember, you are fueling your workouts with food and then using food to help recover afterward. The body cannot perform when it is not properly fueled. Many people don't eat anything before they exercise, and for some people, it works for them. But for others, it is dangerous, especially if they are doing a high-intensity workout.

You should not eat right before your workout. This can cause nausea and stomach distress because once you start exercising, the body shunts the blood to the muscles to provide oxygen and nutrients. As a result, digestion halts, and the person starts to feel sick.

The best time to eat is about one or two hours before a workout, and the preferable choices are foods that get glucose flowing into the bloodstream slowly. Fruit, fruit bars, whole grain toast with peanut butter, oatmeal, or nuts would all be good choices because they have carbohydrates (for energy) and also fiber. Stay away from too much protein or fat because these foods take longer to digest. Can you imagine doing a workout right after you had a huge hamburger?

And there are many people who work out in the morning before they eat anything. This does work for many people—unless the workout is long and intense. Working out before eating first does make your body burn more fat because it does not have glucose readily available after fasting all night.

If that works for you, go ahead and try it, but after your workout, make sure you eat! Within ninety minutes of exercise, your body is more apt to replenish its energy stores. This is the best time to eat starches along with fat and protein. Therefore, the meal you eat right after your workout should be your favorite meal of the day!

Here are some final tips on how to fuel your workouts:

- Food should be viewed as nourishment of the physical body.
- Remember that we are all different in terms of how food affects us. Twenty minutes after you eat, notice how your body feels. If it feels lethargic or not well, it's probably because of what you ate. If you feel great, that food is a keeper!
- Make sure you seek out natural, whole, living foods. This includes fresh fruits, vegetables, beans, nuts, and whole grains.
- If you eat processed foods, start looking at the labels. If you don't recognize an ingredient or know what it is, it is probably a chemical. And chemicals don't fuel your performance. Also, be on the lookout for sugar. Anything that ends in "ase" is a form of sugar.
- Vary your diet and get creative with food and recipes! It can be really fun to come up with meals that are not only healthy but also yummy!
- Remember to seek quality in protein sources and don't eat too much at any meal. The best way to measure protein is to have just what you can fit into your palm. That is usually between 4 and 6 ounces. You don't need more than that at any meal.

- Try to eat at least one large salad a day. Add fresh fruits and veggies. Fruits are your cleaners and vegetables are your restorers. These are your real fuel foods! They also have a lot of fiber and pass through your system quickly. No FOS!

- Practice systematic undereating and stop eating when you are 80 percent full. Overeating causes bloating, gas, heartburn, and interferes with food digestion. You would never load a washing machine up to the top with clothes, so why do that to your stomach?

- Eat slowly. Enjoy your food! Put your fork down between bites to slow down. You might actually eat less. Also, too many people eat too fast and don't even taste their food.

- Remember to drink your water! Carry it with you if you need to have it at work or school or in your car.

- Stay away from fast-food chains. Most of these foods are high in calories, fat, and sugar and low in fiber.

- Limit junk foods such as candies, cookies, doughnuts, French fries, soft drinks, white sugar, and anything with white flour. They will lead to disease, sickness, sluggishness, nervousness, irritability, and constipation.

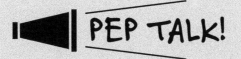

I hope you learned some new things about nutrition that you can incorporate into your lifestyle. Food should be nutritious, delicious and also fuel your body and mind. So take a look at your diet now and see where you can make some positive changes. Remember that it doesn't have to be a perfect plan. Try crowding out foods you know that are unhealthy with more natural whole foods. Also, get creative with food and explore new options. As Jack LaLanne used to say, "Fitness is the King and Nutrition is the Queen. Put them together and you have a Kingdom!"

CHAPTER 9

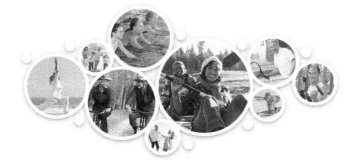

Body Composition—Your Body Doesn't Really Care How Much It Weighs

Weight control and body composition are directly related to each other but they are also distinctly different. *Weight control* refers to maintaining, losing, or gaining weight as indicated by a scale. *Body composition*, on the other hand, refers to how much of your body is either fat or lean body mass. (*Lean body mass* is everything except fat.)

Most people make the mistake of trying to control their weight without knowing their body composition. When you stand on a scale, your total body weight is measured, which is both body fat and lean body mass combined. Since muscle weighs more than fat, it is possible that a person is achieving significant positive body composition changes (more muscle, less fat), while the scale indicates either no difference in weight or even a slight increase.

Frustrating to say the least!

I have seen many people who weigh the same on the scale and are even the same height, but some are fit and others are obese. Weight also fluctuates because of water content in the body. Muscle contains far more water as a percentage of weight than fat tissue (73 percent as compared to 20 percent). Also, muscle burns more calories pound for pound than fat. Replacing a pound of fat with a pound of muscle and continuing to eat the same number of calories will actually cause a person to burn more fat at rest because of the increase in muscle.

Instead of being so concerned about how much we weigh, we should be more concerned about what actually constitutes the weight. I think most people would prefer to have more muscle on their bodies and less fat in order to live their lives to the fullest. If we really want to win the battle of the bulge and lose weight, it would be helpful to know what our body composition is, what a healthy body composition is for us, and how to get there without jeopardizing our health and well-being.

There are no shortcuts to losing weight if you want the weight loss to be a fat loss. Losing stored fat takes time. One pound of fat contains approximately 3,500 calories. There is no way you could possibly lose one pound of fat a day even if you ate nothing and worked out for five hours. But you could lose one pound on the scale, but it would be water loss, which would come back on easily.

Methods for Determining Body Composition

A normal body composition range for a woman is approximately 25 percent body fat while a typical male is 18 percent. Having too much fat on our bodies is a condition called *obesity* and typically starts when a woman has over 30 percent body fat and a male has over 25 percent body fat.

Obesity puts us at risk of many diseases, including heart disease, certain cancers, and type 2 diabetes. Having too little fat on our bodies can cause health problems as well, especially for women. Women who have under 10 percent body fat can experience menstrual irregularities, amenorrhea (cessation of periods not related to menopause), and put themselves at risk for osteoporosis. Therefore, having a healthy body composition is a health priority.

Some of the methods used to determine body composition are discussed in the following sections.

Body Mass Index (BMI)

One tool that is used often but is not accurate for people with a large amount of muscle mass is the *BMI scale*, which many doctors and health insurance companies use. It is an assessment based on height and weight. Anyone with a BMI over 30 on this assessment is considered obese, the range of 25-29 is overweight, 20-24 is normal, and below 20 is underweight.

While it is accurate for most people, a person with above average amounts of muscle will usually test high on this scale and that includes many athletes. I don't think a body builder with 3 percent fat on his body and bulging muscles is obese.

Computed Tomography (CT) and Magnetic Resonance Imaging (MRI)

The most accurate methods to determine obesity are to use *computed tomography (CT)* or *magnetic resonance imaging (MRI)* to measure the amount of visceral fat. These tests are very accurate in assessing health risks from excess amounts of fat that cover the organs, but they are expensive and also require specialized equipment.

Bioelectrical Impedance

This technique is gaining in popularity and is becoming more accurate as technology improves. For the full test, small electrodes are attached to your hands and feet, and the machine sends a signal from one electrode to the other.

Don't worry. You won't get electrocuted or even feel anything.

The faster the signal travels, the more muscle you have. This is because water conducts electricity, and muscles are mostly water. Fat, on the other hand, is only 10-20 percent water, so it impedes or slows down the signal.

The test is fast and painless. A person's hydration may affect the results, so having coffee before the test or drinking alcohol the night before might make the test less accurate in terms of correctly measuring the percentage of fat.

Many health clubs and some hospitals offer this test. There are also bioelectrical impedance options on some scales, but they are not as accurate. I have a portable analyzer I use on my students called the Omron Body Fat-Loss Monitor (www.omronhealthcare.com). While it is not 100 percent accurate, it does give people a great way to track their body composition.

Waist Circumference

This is an easy measurement of the waist at the navel. Since abdominal fat is mostly visceral fat, which is fat around the organs, this is an important measurement for health reasons. If a man has a waist circumference of 40 inches or more he is considered at high risk for health- related problems. A woman is at high risk if her waist circumference is more than 35 inches.

How Do You Lose Body Fat?

The bottom line is to exercise more and eat less. And you have to be patient and also take sugar out of your diet. Remember that sugar in the diet and its effect on insulin causes us to store more fat in our bodies and makes it harder to burn. Believe it or not, losing fat is not hard; it just takes time, and you don't have to do high-intensity exercises to burn fat for fuel.

Think of it as going from a fat-storing machine to a fat-burning machine. Here are some guidelines for changing your body composition:

1. Do not go below 1200 calories a day in your food intake. We need at least this many calories for normal body processes, such as heart function, breathing, and digestion, which all require energy and calories. If you go below 1200 calories, your body will respond by lowering your Basal Metabolic Rate, which is how many calories you burn at rest.

2. Maximum weight loss should be no more than 1-2 pounds a week.

3. Eat more whole foods with fiber and less processed foods with sugar.

4. Include an endurance type program of exercise for 30 minutes at least three days a week at a light to moderate intensity.

5. For even greater results, add resistance training at least twice a week for all the major muscle groups.

6. Increase your activities of daily living and find more reasons to move. Take the stairs instead of the elevator. Walk instead of drive when you can or ride your bike. Remember, we want to turn our bodies into fat-burning machines, not fat-storing machines.

7. Drink a lot of water as it suppresses the appetite and helps the body metabolize stored fat.

8. Stay away from short-term programs, fad diets, or weight-loss supplements. Instead, choose a lifestyle program you can stay with for the rest of your life.

9. Remember to be patient with yourself. It takes time to change body composition.

10. Stay away from fast-food restaurants and processed foods.

11. Remember that your progress will be unique to you. Everyone's bodies respond to changes differently.

Visualize yourself at the body composition you want to be. Actually see this in your mind. One of my friends put up a picture of herself when she was at her "best self" when she was younger. Another friend combined a photo of her face with a picture of a model's body. Even though she might not eventually get that body, it is something to strive for and move toward.

The Weight-Loss Industry

Notice I didn't say the Body Composition Industry. If you want to lose weight, there are lots of people out there who are ready and willing to help. In fact, the weight loss industry is a billion-dollar industry but with only a 2 percent success rate. Usually 98 percent of the people who lose weight with these programs regain the weight they lost and even put on more. The main reason for this is that these programs are short term and don't teach lifelong lifestyle skills. Also, they focus on losing weight as measured by the scale, not changing body composition.

Weight-loss clinics are everywhere, and we see them advertised all the time. While some people do have success, many people don't, and what they usually end up losing is a lot of money instead of fat.

Remember that pounds can drop from the scale rapidly and that weight loss is mostly water. So people do lose weight, but most cannot sustain the weight loss because these programs are not lifetime eating plans. Most of these programs do not even emphasize exercise, and some of these centers also prescribe weight-loss supplements.

Most diets fail because they inspire rebellion. They focus on what you can't eat rather than what you should eat. If you told me I could never have chocolate again, I would probably feel deprived and not want to stay on your plan for very long. Who could live without chocolate?

The key is to say *no* to dieting. People who are successful at losing fat and keeping it off permanently have an eating plan that works for them and fuels their life and goals, and they have an exercise program that is a priority in their lives. They are not obsessed about weight or food; they are too busy enjoying their lives. They don't restrict themselves or feel deprived. They use common sense when it comes to their food choices and do splurge at times. But most of what they eat is healthy. They don't eat unless they are hungry and stop before they are full and rely on internal regulation rather than external regulation.

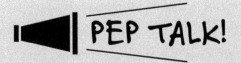

So, if you are serious about losing weight, get on board for the long haul and remember that quick fixes don't work. If you take it slow and change your eating habits and exercise, you will feel so good that you might not even notice the changes in your body composition, but they will come. And don't wait until you lose weight to start living! Live the life you plan on living when you lose the weight, now! You will be surprised at how easy it is to make positive lifestyle changes that lead to having a healthy body composition for life. Most people who do have healthy body compositions are not consumed by restrictive dieting. They are too busy enjoying their lives!

CHAPTER 10

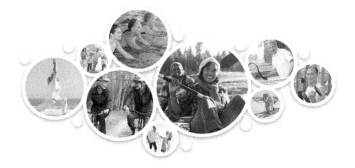

Stress Management

"**A**nyone stressed out?"

When I ask this question in my class, most of the hands go up. Most of us have stress in our lives, and that is normal. The simplest definition of *stress* is *how we respond to CHANGE.*

Being able to take on the challenges of life is important to achieving overall health. Exercise as a stress management tool has been shown to be very effective in helping people manage a stressful life. But for many people, it is not enough. Does it surprise you to know that between 70 and 90 percent of visits to doctors are stress related? Since no one can live a stress-free life, learning how to manage stress is imperative for everyone who wants to achieve optimal health.

In itself, stress is neither positive nor negative. *It is our reactions to stress* that can either be positive or negative, and these responses become the habits that lead us either to personal growth or mental debilitation. We can't control everything that happens to us, but we can always control how we respond.

Therein lies our power.

We all need a certain amount of stress to be healthy and for us to achieve personal growth. However, most of us let too much stress into our lives, and most of it is preventable because the source of most of our stress is in our minds.

Fight or Flight Syndrome

All animals, including humans, are physiologically equipped to deal with stress. It is called the *flight or fight response,* and it basically gets the body ready to either fight or run away. This is a survival mechanism.

Imagine you are walking down a dark, empty street late at night by yourself. Halfway down the street someone comes toward you. If you perceive this as a threat, your body responds to this situation with the fight or flight syndrome. The physiological changes elicited by this survival mechanism are: breathing becomes fast and shallow, the heart beats faster, muscles tense up, pupils and bronchioles dilate, blood pressure rises, glucose and fatty acids and adrenaline are released into the blood.

In this situation, if the person approaching you was an actual threat, your body is prepared to respond to either fight off the offender or escape. If the person is not a threat and just walks past you, your body was put in this heightened state for nothing, and if this response happens too often, the result is a physical wear and tear on the body, which can ultimately cause disease and even death.

Situations that call for the fight or flight response are those that are life-threatening. A car coming at you at 80 miles an hour is obviously a life-threatening situation. I call these *legitimate stressors*.

But in modern life, most of the events that throw us out of *homeostasis* (biological balance or equilibrium) are not *legitimate*. An argument, a person calling you a name, job stresses, losing a game, money problems, relationship challenges, health challenges, etc. all are examples of changes that should not activate the fight or flight response. But unfortunately, they can, and it happens way too often. I call these stressors, which do not threaten our survival, *neurotic stressors*, and the good news is that we can control most of these stressors by changing our perceptions.

Most modern-day stressors are not caused by *physical* events. Instead, they are *psychological*, and our power to manage stress is also in our minds. *We do NOT have to be victims when it comes to stress.* In fact, if we viewed some of these stressors in a more positive light, they can actually help lead us to success.

The Stress Model

The *stress model* follows a progression of when a person first recognizes a stressor to the actual health consequences. The sooner a person intervenes in this progression, the better in terms of the outcome.

Stressor
  Perception of the Event
    Emotional Response
      Physiological Response
        Health Consequence

Stressors—Getting to Know Them

Most of us know what causes stress in our lives. Many of these stressors are predictable and avoidable. If you know that traffic causes you a great deal of stress, you can probably avoid it by either leaving at a different time or taking a different route. If a person annoys you a great deal, try to avoid situations where you will have to deal with this person. In other words, you don't have to "reach out and touch" a stressor that is avoidable unless you choose to do so.

Reducing sources of stress is an effective means of lowering the impact of stress in your life. Identify which sources of stress are unnecessary and try to eliminate those activities. With predictable stress, you usually have time to plan.

Creating roadblocks to this first stage of the stress model can eliminate many of our everyday stressors. And also, for people who find they are doing too much for others, saying NO is a good word to have at the tip of your tongue.

Perception of the Event

Once you have identified a stressor, unless it is immediately life threatening, you have a choice as to how you want to view it; that is, the meaning that you attach to the stressor is totally within your control. One helpful tool in stopping stressors at this stage is to use *selective awareness*. In other words, try to focus on the positive aspects of the situation instead of the negative ones. Remember, before you feel anything from a neurotic stressor, you must first attach a meaning to it. And most of us react too quickly to something negative.

The following is an example of using selective awareness:

Stressor	**Negative Perception**
Argument with husband	He hates me and doesn't love me anymore.

In this example, the stressor is not life threatening—it is just words. The meaning is very negative and probably blown out of proportion. If this negative perception is attached to the stressor, the emotions felt will probably also be negative: sad, mad, and depressed. And as we know, emotions can take a toll on our physical health.

Now, let's change the perception:

Stressor	**Positive Perception**
Argument with husband	We have our own ideas; we are not going to agree all the time.

With the second example, which might have taken a little more time to come up with, instead of feeling sad, mad, and depressed, the person will probably feel empowered and energized and actually have a positive mind-body response instead of a negative one.

When I share this example with my students, they say that it's too easy and everyone can do this if they want. My response to them is usually, yes it is—so why don't we do it?

Remember that we all have the ability to attach whatever meaning we want to any stressor. It is always our choice as to how we want to view a situation or a challenge. *We are **not** victims of stress! We have more control than we realize!*

Emotional Response

If we don't stop the stress at the first or second stage of the stress response, then we have to learn to deal with our emotions. The two most common stress emotions are anger and fear, which can ultimately lead to depression. The average person has at least ten episodes of anger or fear during a typical day, so they are not unusual.

Standing in lines, inconsiderate drivers, and poor service are just a few examples of everyday hassles that fuel these emotions. Relaxation techniques, meditation, and deep-breathing exercises help to deal with stressful emotions. That's one reason why so many people are turning to yoga to help deal with stress.

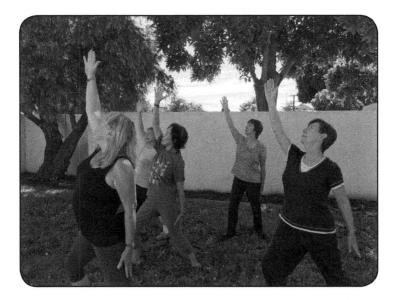

Also, learning how to cope with your emotions is a key to making them work for you. If you allow the anger in, what are you going to do about it? Instead of allowing anger to punish you with its intensity, use the energy to do something about the situation that caused it. If you can properly channel your anger, you might be motivated to make some major changes in your life. But unresolved anger is very dangerous to your health.

Physiological Response

The *physiological response* is what happens to the body as a result of unmanaged stress. There is a very strong mind-body response, and your body does start to give signals when it is being compromised by too much stress.

Exercise is usually a great stress reliever at any part of the stress response but is especially important at this stage. Exercise helps to break down the stress hormones, clear the blood of the excess glucose and fatty acids of the fight or flight response, and also promotes the secretion of endorphins in the brain, which are the body's natural opiates. Also, endorphins relieve pain and elevate mood. So exercise as a stress reliever is a very powerful way to keep from getting sick.

Health Consequences

Hopefully, you will not get this far down on the stress progression. However, most doctors are now aware of the connection between stress and illness and usually will write a prescription if they can for most of the health consequences, unless they require surgery or other types of treatment. This is what they are trained to do. They are not responsible for what got you to this place—you are!

Once you understand what stress is and how it progresses, you should be more equipped to deal with stress in all its forms. Remember, the sooner you intervene in the stress progression, the better chance you have of staying healthy.

Here is a list of popular stress management tools. We are all different in what works for us, so try out the ones that you want to do.

- View stress as a challenge instead of a problem. Remember that each problem is either an opportunity to grow and learn or an obstacle to keep you from growing and learning. You get to make the choice.

- Take responsibility for your choices. Projecting blame or making excuses keeps you stuck and is an ineffective defense mechanism. Only when you are accountable are you powerful. Remember that you can't change other people or what has happened in the past, so control what you can, that is, *your* choices and *your* attitudes.
- Think before you act. My husband always says: "The quality of your choices determines the quality of your life. Choose wisely."
- Learn to say, "NO." Stop taking on projects that you are not passionate about.
- Ask for help if you need it. There are many people and organizations that are there just to help us get through life's challenges. You never have to go at it alone unless you really want to. It is not shameful or weak to ask for help.
- Schedule time for *yourself*. Find time each day to relax or do something you enjoy. Remember that taking an occasional break from your work is not wasting time. In fact, it will improve your overall productivity and reenergize you.

Even with stress management tools, it is impossible to eliminate all forms of stress from our daily lives. Therefore, it becomes necessary to know some stress relievers to reduce the harmful effects of stress. Find one or several you think might work for you.

1. Remember to exercise. Any type of exercise works as long as you enjoy it and are consistent. Just don't do too much too soon or over train. You don't want your stress reliever to become a source of stress, and you don't want to injure yourself.

2. Take a vacation. Even if it's a "staycation." Change your surroundings and go someplace new.

3. Get a massage. If you have never had one, just do it!

4. Read books for enjoyment.

5. Listen to music you enjoy.

6. Take up a new hobby.

7. Get a pet. They are wonderful sources of unconditional love.

8. Use humor. Smile and laugh every day.

9. Keep a journal. Writing down your feelings is a great way to get them out of your head.

10. Cut down on foods that you know are unhealthy, especially sugar, alcohol, and junk food.

11. Develop a support system. Having friends and family are important for managing stress. Make sure you keep in touch with the people who care about you. They are golden!

12. Give yourself a moment of silence each day. Put down your cell phone and get off the computer and turn off the "fake" news.

13. Practice mindfulness by living in the present moment. Feeling guilty about the past or worrying about the future is a major waste of time.

14. Let go of resentments and forgive if possible. Resentment is like taking poison and hoping it will kill someone else. Forgiving is a gift you give to yourself, not another person. And what's cool is that the other person doesn't even have to know that you forgave him or her!

15. Take a moment every day to appreciate what you have. A great practice is to write in a journal at night everything you are grateful for that happened that day. We all have so many

things in our lives that are precious. Instead of focusing on what is wrong, look for the good and you will find it.

16. Give to others without expecting anything back.

17. Volunteer if you can or become a mentor.

18. Call or write an old friend if you haven't been in touch for a while.

19. Get outside and enjoy nature. Sometimes, just a walk along the beach, in the forest, or in a park is just what the doctor ordered.

20. Clean up clutter. The more stuff you have around you, the less energy you have. So start to clear it out. Give away anything you have not used lately to someone who will use it and appreciate it. There are several social media platforms where you can sell your items online such as Ebay and Let Go. Get the apps on your phone and get rid of both your stuff and your stress.

21. Make sure you also get your sleep. This is one of the best stress management tools. Individual needs vary in terms of how much is needed, but most people need at least seven hours to feel their best. When you sleep, your body is recovering and regenerating.

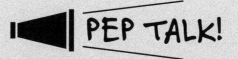

Remember that no one is immune to stress. Only the dead have no stress. Your challenge is not to avoid all stressors, but to learn how to live with stressors in your life. It is never the type of stress or even the amount that makes you different from anyone else. The difference is how you perceive the stressors and choose to deal with them. And a fit lifestyle is one of the best stress management tools you can have in your toolbox. So keep moving!

CHAPTER 11

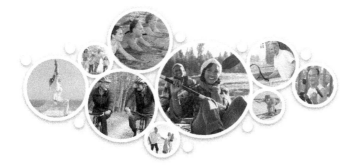

Staying Fit for Life

We cannot store fitness. Therefore, if we want to stay fit and enjoy our life to the fullest, we need to make exercise and fitness an integral part of our lifestyle. Too often, people drop out of a fitness program because they are unmotivated or because they don't see results fast enough.

We do live in the land of the "quick fix" where we want everything now, and if we don't get what we want, when we want it, we quit. We also tend to focus on our bodies' imperfections instead of looking at the whole picture of what a fit lifestyle offers.

I think most of us want to be disease-free and have the energy and physical capacity to live our lives to the fullest.

I know that's what I want.

I also don't want to have my health decline as I get older as I see so often in our society. We are living longer, but as a whole, not better. I want my second half of life to be as awesome as the first, and maybe even better! Don't YOU?

So how can we stay motivated to work out for the rest of our lives? First of all, we must shut off the TV, click off the computer, stop playing video games, stop watching soap operas and talk shows. Do we really just want to observe life, or do we want to live it?

I think most of us want to live it fully all the way to the end. Where do I sign up to live long and die short? Exercise is definitely a key. Buy some new exercise shoes, get outside and enjoy the sun, fresh air, and blue skies; enjoy the fact that you can move your body!

And never take your amazing body for granted.

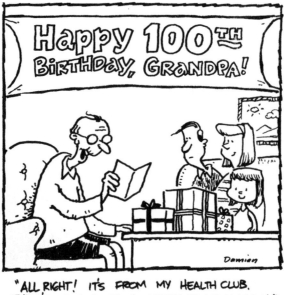

"ALL RIGHT! IT'S FROM MY HEALTH CLUB. THEY'VE GIVEN ME A LIFETIME MEMERSHIP!"

Here are some tips on how to keep fitness a fun part of your lifestyle for as long as you are alive:

- Make the commitment to exercise because you want to do something for *you*. If you are healthy and happy, then you can also help others in your life. But if you are not at your best, then you cannot be of much use to others. So take care of YOU.
- Remember to pick activities that you enjoy. Exercise is not a punishment. It should also make you feel great and be safe.
- When you are working out, enjoy the moment. Keep negative thoughts out of your mind when you exercise. This is YOUR time!
- Remember that variety is the spice of life. Add new activities and exercises periodically to spice up your workouts. There is never any reason to be bored unless you want to be.
- Replace negative incentives with positive ones. Focus on what you want out of your exercise program instead of what you don't want.
- Make excuses to be more active instead of less active. Walk whenever you can. Never sit for more than an hour at a time. Take the stairs instead of the elevators or escalators. Ride your bike to work instead of driving. Increasing the activities of daily living is a great way to get more positive results from working out. It all counts!
- A workout partner can help you get motivated and keep you accountable. Plus, working out is usually more fun when you do it with someone else. And if you want to improve your social life, get active with a group!
- Reinforce your efforts. Reward yourself for reaching both long-term and mini-goals.
- Exercise outside as much as possible. Sunlight tends to

improve mood. You'll also get to absorb the "sunshine vitamin, vitamin D."

- Pick a fit role model that you know and find out what his or her secrets are to keeping fit and happy.

- Do not weigh yourself more than once every two weeks. The scale as you know does not really show what is going on in your body. You could be getting great results, but the scale might not show any changes. Remember that muscle weighs more than fat, and you want the muscle!

- Avoid negative people who do not support your new lifestyle. They are usually jealous because they are too lazy to work out and want to sabotage your efforts so they have more company in the "unfit, woe is me society."

- See yourself as a fit individual and live the lifestyle. Don't wait until you reach your goal to start enjoying life to the fullest. Remember, this is a life journey, not a destination.

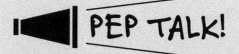

Regular exercise really is the closest thing to the fountain of youth. People who work out are physiologically and psychologically younger than their sedentary friends. Most of the symptoms of aging are caused by inactivity, not chronological age. If you don't want to get old or are looking to turn back the clock, now is the time to make exercise a part of your routine. You wouldn't think of going days without brushing your teeth, would you? And just because other people have accepted being over the hill doesn't mean that you have to do the same.

The second half of life really can be the best half, but it's up to you. Promise yourself to make fitness and movement an integral and enjoyable part of your lifestyle. If you are having fun getting fit, your overall life might also become more fun since you will have the energy and physical ability to do more of the activities that you enjoy. I am confident you will notice a huge difference in your overall health and feel rejuvenated and happier. A fit mind and body is definitely an advantage to withstand the demands of life and also help you enjoy your life to the fullest regardless of age. Don't you owe it to yourself to make that happen for YOU?

So what are you waiting for? Get MOVING today!

Additional Resources

Where to Go for More Information

AMERICAN SENIOR FITNESS ASSOCIATION

- Since 1992, the leader in older adult fitness education
- www.seniorfitness.net

AARP

- Healthy Living – Fitness, Nutrition, Wellness
- AARP's **Healthy Living** channel provides news and information on fitness, nutrition, and wellness.
- www.aarp.org/health/healthy-living

IDEA

- Health and Fitness Association
- Great articles and fitness certifications.
- http://www.ideafit.com/home

PREVENTION

- Articles on health, fitness, and diet.
- http://www.prevention.com

NEXT AVENUE

- "Where grown-ups keep growing."
- http://www.nextavenue.org

SIXTY AND ME

- A site for women over sixty with inspiring articles and stories.
- http://sixtyandme.com

BOOMER FITNESS

- Boomer Fitness is a team of fitness and nutrition experts who strive to create powerful and engaging fitness and wellness programs for the Baby Boomer Generation.
- www.boomerfitness.com

WOMEN OVER 50

- Great advice and articles for women.
- https://betterafter50.com

SUPER SENIOR FITNESS; GETTING OLD IS NOT FOR WEAKLINGS

- Ron Krayewski, a personal trainer of senior fitness and strength-training exercises, shares health tips and fun activities.
- www.superseniorfitness.com

SENIORITY HEALTH

- A great site for men over 40.
- https://seniorityhealth.com

EVERYTHING ZOOMER

- Fun Canadian website for people over 45—Zoomers! Everything from health, diet, lifestyle to travel and money. Also some great articles about inspirational seniors. It can make your day!
- www.everythingzoomer.com

BOOMERS LIFE

- http://www.boomerslife.org
- One of the most popular Baby Boomer sites on the web. Covers music, people, health, and other issues of interest to Boomers. Plus, it has links to many other Boomer websites! You can't help but smile when you visit this site! So COOL!

About the Author

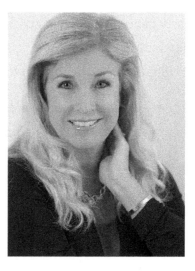

Sharkie Zartman is a former USA All-American volleyball athlete and champion competitor at UCLA where her jersey was retired. She was a member of the U.S. Women's National Volleyball Team and also competed in the Women's Professional Beach Volleyball Association for five years and is a member of the California Beach Volleyball Hall of Fame.

As a coach, Sharkie led El Camino College to nine league and two state volleyball titles, and with her husband, Pat, she helped the South Bay Spoilers club team win multiple national titles.

Sharkie holds a B.S. in Kinesiology and an M.S. in Instructional Technology. She has taught health and fitness at the community college level for over forty years and has brought innovative fitness programs into the college curriculum. She taught and coached thousands of students and athletes and was honored with both coaching and instructional awards. She hosts "Sharkie's Pep Talk" on Healthy Life.Net Radio and has interviewed hundreds of holistic health and fitness experts from around the globe. Sharkie is a certified health coach with the official sanction of the New York State Education Department and the Institute of Integrative Nutrition.

Her passion and mission is helping people take an empowered approach to life and aging so they can have optimal health and success at any age. She lives in Hermosa Beach with her husband Pat.

Sharkie has authored five books, including:

- *Take on Aging as a Sport; The Athletic Approach to Aging*
- *Shark Sense, Getting in Touch with Your Inner Shark*
- *So You Think You Can Coach Kids?*
- *Youth Volleyball; The Guide for Coaches and Parents*

Visit her on www.sharkiezartman.com
Facebook: Take on Aging as a Sport